T0226718

Hypogonadism

Editor

JOSEPH P. ALUKAL

UROLOGIC CLINICS OF NORTH AMERICA

www.urologic.theclinics.com

Consulting Editor
SAMIR S. TANEJA

May 2016 • Volume 43 • Number 2

ELSEVIER

1600 John F. Kennedy Boulevard • Suite 1800 • Philadelphia, Pennsylvania, 19103-2899

http://www.theclinics.com

UROLOGIC CLINICS OF NORTH AMERICA Volume 43, Number 2
May 2016 ISSN 0094-0143, ISBN-13: 978-0-323-44483-5

Editor: Kerry Holland
Developmental Editor: Alison Swety

Urologic Clinics of North America (ISSN 0094-0143) is published quarterly by Elsevier Inc., 360 Park Avenue South, New York, NY 10010-1710. Months of issue are February, May, August, and November. Business and Editorial Offices: 1600 John F. Kennedy Blvd., Suite 1800, Philadelphia, PA 19103-2899. Periodicals postage paid at New York, NY and additional mailing offices. Subscription prices are $360.00 per year (US individuals), $660.00 per year (US institutions), $415.00 per year (Canadian individuals), $825.00 per year (Canadian institutions), $515.00 per year (foreign individuals), and $825.00 per year (foreign institutions). Foreign air speed delivery is included in all *Clinics* subscription prices. All prices are subject to change without notice. **POSTMASTER:** Send address changes to *Urologic Clinics of North America*, Elsevier Health Sciences Division, Subscription Customer Service, 3251 Riverport Lane, Maryland Heights, MO 63043. **Customer Service: 1-800-654-2452 (US). From outside the United States, call 1-314-447-8871. Fax: 1-314-447-8029. E-mail: JournalsCustomerServiceusa@elsevier.com (for print support)** and **JournalsOnlineSupport-usa@elsevier.com (for online support)**.

Reprints. For copies of 100 or more, of articles in this publication, please contact the Commercial Reprints Department, Elsevier Inc., 360 Park Avenue South, New York, New York 10010-1710. Tel.: 212-633-3874; Fax: 212-633-3820; E-mail: reprints@elsevier.com.

Urologic Clinics of North America is covered in MEDLINE/PubMed (*Index Medicus*), *Excerpta Medica*, *Current Contents/Clinical Medicine*, *Science Citation Index*, and *ISI/BIOMED*.

PROGRAM OBJECTIVE

The goal of *Urologic Clinics of North America* is to keep practicing urologists and urology residents up to date with current clinical practice in urology by providing timely articles reviewing the state of the art in patient care.

TARGET AUDIENCE

Practicing urologists, urology residents and other health care professionals practicing in the discipline of urology.

LEARNING OBJECTIVES

Upon completion of this activity, participants will be able to:
1. Review the physiology and diagnosis of male hypogonadism.
2. Discuss testosterone treatment and prescription in the management of hypogonadism.
3. Recognize the role of testosterone deficiency in sexual function, sleep apnea, and prostate function.

ACCREDITATION

The Elsevier Office of Continuing Medical Education (EOCME) is accredited by the Accreditation Council for Continuing Medical Education (ACCME) to provide continuing medical education for physicians.

The EOCME designates this enduring material for a maximum of 15 *AMA PRA Category 1 Credit*(s)™. Physicians should claim only the credit commensurate with the extent of their participation in the activity.

All other health care professionals requesting continuing education credit for this enduring material will be issued a certificate of participation.

DISCLOSURE OF CONFLICTS OF INTEREST

The EOCME assesses conflict of interest with its instructors, faculty, planners, and other individuals who are in a position to control the content of CME activities. All relevant conflicts of interest that are identified are thoroughly vetted by EOCME for fair balance, scientific objectivity, and patient care recommendations. EOCME is committed to providing its learners with CME activities that promote improvements or quality in healthcare and not a specific proprietary business or a commercial interest.

The planning committee, staff, authors and editors listed below have identified no financial relationships or relationships to products or devices they or their spouse/life partner have with commercial interest related to the content of this CME activity:

Joseph P. Alukal, MD; Rohan Bansal, BA; Jeffery S. Berger, MD; Omar Burschtin, MD; Cenk Cengiz, BS; Aaron Chidakel, MD; Patricia Freitas Corradi, MD; Renato B. Corradi, MD; Emily Davidson, BS; Michael L. Eisenberg, MD; Anjali Fortna; Joseph Scott Gabrielsen, MD, PhD; John R. Gannon, MD; Eugenia Gianos, MD; Loren Wissner Greene, MD, MA, FACE, FACP; Russell P. Hayden, MD; Amin S. Herati, MD; Kerry Holland; Indu Kumari; Dolores J. Lamb, PhD; Steven Lamm, MD; Herbert Lepor, MD; Mark C. Lindgren, MD; Bobby B. Najari, MD; Samuel J. Ohlander, MD; Anna Ross, MD; Arthur Schwartzbard, MD; Megan Suermann; Monique S. Tanna, MD; Cigdem Tanrikut, MD, FACS; Thomas J. Walsh, MD, MS; Jing Wang, MD.

The planning committee, staff, authors and editors listed below have identified financial relationships or relationships to products or devices they or their spouse/life partner have with commercial interest related to the content of this CME activity:

Shalender Bhasin, MB, BS is a consultant/advisor for AbbVie, Inc.; Eli Lilly and Company; Novartis AG; and Sanofi, has stock ownership in FPT, LLC, and has research support from AbbVie, Inc.; Eli Lily and Company; Regeneron Pharmaceuticals, Inc.; and Transition Therapeutics Inc.

Mohit Khera, MD, MBA, MPH is a consultant/advisor for AbbVie, Inc.; Endo Pharmaceuticals Inc.; Lipocine Inc.; and Repros Therapeutics Inc.

Larry I. Lipshultz, MD is on the speakers' bureau for Boston Scientific Company or its affiliates and Repros Therapeutics Inc., is a consultant/advisor for Boston Scientific Company or its affiliates; Endo Pharmaceuticals Inc.; Repros Therapeutics Inc.; and AbbVie, Inc., and has research support from Endo Pharmaceuticals Inc. and Repros Therapeutics Inc.

Abraham Morgentaler, MD is on the speakers' bureau for Bayer AG; Lipocine Inc.; and Pfizer Inc., is a consultant/advisor for AbbVie, Inc.; Clarus Ventures, LLC; Endo Pharmaceuticals Inc.; and TesoRx LLC, and has research support from Eli Lily and Company and Endo Pharmaceuticals Inc.

Samir S. Taneja, MD is a consultant/advisor for Bayer AG; Eigen Pharma LLC; GTx, Inc.; HealthTronics, Inc.; and Hitachi, Ltd.

James Underberg, MD is on the speakers' bureau for Merck & Co., Inc.; Amgen Inc; Alexion; Regeneron Pharmaceuticals, Inc.; and AstraZeneca, is a consultant/advisor for Akcea Therapeutics; Amgen Inc; Sanofi; Alexion; Amarin Corporation; and Recombine, and has research support from Pfizer Inc. and Aegerion Pharmaceuticals, Inc.

Howard S. Weintraub, MD, FACC is on the speakers' bureau for Amarin Corporation; Amgen Inc; and Bristol-Myers Squibb Company, is a consultant/advisor for Amgen Inc; Gilead; and Sanofi, and has research support from Amarin Corporation and Sanofi.

UNAPPROVED/OFF-LABEL USE DISCLOSURE

The EOCME requires CME faculty to disclose to the participants:

1. When products or procedures being discussed are off-label, unlabelled, experimental, and/or investigational (not US Food and Drug Administration [FDA] approved); and
2. Any limitations on the information presented, such as data that are preliminary or that represent ongoing research, interim analyses, and/or unsupported opinions. Faculty may discuss information about pharmaceutical agents that is outside of FDA-approved labelling. This information is intended solely for CME and is not intended to promote off-label use of these medications. If you have any questions, contact the medical affairs department of the manufacturer for the most recent prescribing information.

TO ENROLL

To enroll in the *Urologic Clinics of North America* Continuing Medical Education program, call customer service at 1-800-654-2452 or sign up online at http://www.theclinics.com/home/cme. The CME program is available to subscribers for an additional annual fee of USD $270.

METHOD OF PARTICIPATION

In order to claim credit, participants must complete the following:

1. Complete enrolment as indicated above.
2. Read the activity.
3. Complete the CME Test and Evaluation. Participants must achieve a score of 70% on the test. All CME Tests and Evaluations must be completed online.

CME INQUIRIES/SPECIAL NEEDS

For all CME inquiries or special needs, please contact elsevierCME@elsevier.com.

Contributors

CONSULTING EDITOR

SAMIR S. TANEJA, MD
The James M. Neissa and Janet Riha Neissa
Professor of Urologic Oncology; Professor of
Urology and Radiology; Director, Division of
Urologic Oncology; Co-Director, Department
of Urology, Smilow Comprehensive Prostate
Cancer Center, NYU Langone Medical Center,
New York, New York

EDITOR

JOSEPH P. ALUKAL, MD
Director, Male Reproductive Health; Clinical
Assistant Professor, Departments of Urology,
Obstetrics/Gynecology, New York University
School of Medicine, New York, New York

AUTHORS

JOSEPH P. ALUKAL, MD
Director, Male Reproductive Health; Clinical
Assistant Professor, Departments of Urology,
Obstetrics/Gynecology, New York University
School of Medicine, New York, New York

ROHAN BANSAL, BA
Department of Medicine, NYU Langone
Preston Robert Tisch Center for Men's
Health, New York, New York

JEFFERY S. BERGER, MD
Division of Cardiology, New York University
School of Medicine, New York, New York

SHALENDER BHASIN, MB, BS
Director, Research Program in Men's Health:
Aging and Metabolism; Director, The Center for
Clinical Investigation, Brigham and Women's
Hospital, Professor of Medicine, Harvard
Medical School, Boston, Massachusetts

OMAR BURSCHTIN, MD
Associate Professor, Mount Sinai School of
Medicine, Division of Pulmonary, Critical Care
and Sleep Medicine, New York, New York

CENK CENGIZ, BS
Laboratory Technician, Scott Department of
Urology, Center for Reproductive Medicine,
Baylor College of Medicine, Houston, Texas

AARON CHIDAKEL, MD
Clinical Assistant Professor, Department
of Medicine, NYU Langone Preston Robert
Tisch Center for Men's Health, New York,
New York

PATRICIA FREITAS CORRADI, MD
Division of Endocrinology, New York
University School of Medicine, New York,
New York

RENATO B. CORRADI, MD
Urology Service, Department of Surgery,
Memorial Sloan Kettering Cancer Center,
New York, New York

EMILY DAVIDSON, BS
Men's Health Boston, Department of Surgery
(Urology), Harvard Medical School, Chestnut
Hill, Massachusetts

MICHAEL L. EISENBERG, MD
Director, Male Reproductive Medicine and Surgery, Departments of Urology and Obstetrics and Gynecology, Stanford University School of Medicine, Stanford, California

JOSEPH SCOTT GABRIELSEN, MD, PhD
Resident, Department of Urology, Massachusetts General Hospital, Boston, Massachusetts

JOHN R. GANNON, MD
Intermountain Urologic Institute, Intermountain Health Care, Salt Lake City, Utah

EUGENIA GIANOS, MD
Division of Cardiology, New York University School of Medicine, New York, New York

LOREN WISSNER GREENE, MD, MA, FACE, FACP
Clinical Professor of Medicine (Endocrinology) and Obstetrics and Gynecology, Associate Faculty, Bioethics and Medical Ethics, New York University School of Medicine, New York, New York

RUSSELL P. HAYDEN, MD
Department of Urology, Massachusetts General Hospital, Harvard Medical School, Boston, Massachusetts

AMIN S. HERATI, MD
Fellow in Male Infertility and Reproductive Medicine, Scott Department of Urology, Center for Reproductive Medicine, Baylor College of Medicine, Houston, Texas

MOHIT KHERA, MD, MBA, MPH
Associate Professor of Urology, Baylor College of Medicine, Houston, Texas

DOLORES J. LAMB, PhD
Scott Department of Urology, Director of Center for Reproductive Medicine, Vice-Chairman for Research (Urology), Professor of Urology, Professor of Molecular and Cellular Biology, Baylor College of Medicine, Houston, Texas

STEVEN LAMM, MD
Clinical Professor, Department of Medicine, Medical Director; NYU Langone Preston Robert Tisch Center for Men's Health, New York, New York

HERBERT LEPOR, MD
Professor and Chairman, Department of Urology, New York University School of Medicine, New York, New York

MARK C. LINDGREN, MD
Fellow, Division of Male Reproductive Medicine and Surgery, Scott Department of Urology, Baylor College of Medicine, Houston, Texas

LARRY I. LIPSHULTZ, MD
Professor of Urology, Lester and Sue Smith Chair in Reproductive Medicine, Chief, Division of Male Reproductive Medicine and Surgery, Scott Department of Urology, Baylor College of Medicine, Houston, Texas

ABRAHAM MORGENTALER, MD
Men's Health Boston, Department of Surgery (Urology), Harvard Medical School, Chestnut Hill, Massachusetts

BOBBY B. NAJARI, MD
Fellow in Male Reproductive Medicine and Microsurgery, Department of Urology, Weill Cornell Medical College, New York, New York

SAMUEL J. OHLANDER, MD
Fellow, Division of Male Reproductive Medicine and Surgery, Scott Department of Urology, Baylor College of Medicine, Houston, Texas

ANNA ROSS, MD
Research Program in Men's Health: Aging and Metabolism, Brigham and Women's Hospital, Boston, Massachusetts

ARTHUR SCHWARTZBARD, MD
Division of Cardiology, New York University School of Medicine, New York, New York

MONIQUE S. TANNA, MD
Division of Cardiology, New York University School of Medicine, New York, New York

CIGDEM TANRIKUT, MD, FACS
Department of Urology, Massachusetts General Hospital; Assistant Professor of Surgery (Urology), Harvard Medical School, Boston, Massachusetts

JAMES UNDERBERG, MD
Division of Cardiology, New York
University School of Medicine, New York,
New York

THOMAS J. WALSH, MD, MS
Department of Urology, University of
Washington, Seattle, Washington

JING WANG, MD
Sleep Medicine Fellow, NYU School of
Medicine, Division of Pulmonary, Critical Care,
and Sleep Medicine, New York, New York

HOWARD S. WEINTRAUB, MD, FACC
Division of Cardiology, New York University
School of Medicine, New York, New York

Contents

improvement is difficult to measure and seems to differ based on the baseline hormonal status of the patient at the beginning of treatment.

Testosterone and Varicocele   223

Russell P. Hayden and Cigdem Tanrikut

Varicocele is defined as an excessive dilation of the pampiniform plexus. The association between varicocele and infertility has been well-established as evidenced by negative effects on spermatogenesis. Accumulating evidence now suggests that varicocele presents a pantesticular insult, with resultant impairment of Leydig cell function. The presence of a varicocele has been linked to lower serum testosterone levels and varicocelectomy may reverse some of the adverse effects on androgen production. In this article, the evidence linking varicoceles to impaired steroidogenesis and which cohorts of men may benefit most from varicocele repair are discussed.

Testosterone Deficiency and Sleep Apnea   233

Omar Burschtin and Jing Wang

Obstructive sleep apnea (OSA) is a common condition among middle-aged men and is often associated with reduced testosterone (T) levels. OSA can contribute to fatigue and sexual dysfunction in men. There is suggestion that T supplementation alters ventilatory responses, possibly through effects on central chemoreceptors. Traditionally, it has been recommended that T replacement therapy (TRT) be avoided in the presence of untreated severe sleep apnea. With OSA treatment, however, TRT may not only improve hypogonadism, but may also alleviate erectile/sexual dysfunction.

Obesity and Hypogonadism   239

Steven Lamm, Aaron Chidakel, and Rohan Bansal

The relationship between obesity and hypogonadism is complicated. The relationship is bidirectional and there are numerous causative and correlative factors on both sides of the equation. Obesity is increasing in prevalence in epidemic proportions. Likewise, we are beginning to see the rapid increase in the incidence of male hypogonadism. It is only recently that we are learning the ways in which these 2 conditions exacerbate each other, and we are only beginning to understand how by treating one of these conditions, we can help to treat the other as well.

Management of Hypogonadism in Cardiovascular Patients: What Are the Implications of Testosterone Therapy on Cardiovascular Morbidity?   247

Monique S. Tanna, Arthur Schwartzbard, Jeffery S. Berger, James Underberg, Eugenia Gianos, and Howard S. Weintraub

Testosterone replacement therapy is recommended for men with clinical androgen deficiency with decades of evidence supporting its use for treatment of sexual, physical, and psychological consequences of male hypogonadism. In this updated review, the authors discuss the implications of testosterone deficiency and conflicting evidence regarding testosterone replacement therapy and its effects on the cardiovascular system. Based on mounting evidence, the authors conclude that testosterone therapy can be safely considered in men with appropriately diagnosed clinical androgen deficiency and concurrent cardiovascular risk factors and even manifest cardiovascular disease after a thorough discussion of potential risks and with guideline-recommended safety monitoring.

Testosterone supplementation therapy (TST) has become increasingly popular since the turn of the century. Most prescriptions in the U.S. are written by primary care providers, endocrinologists, or urologists. The FDA has requested that pharmaceutical companies provide more long term data on efficacy and safety of testosterone products. Results from these studies will help define the appropriate population for TST going forward. It is hoped that these data combined with physician and public education will minimize inappropriate prescribing and allow those likely to benefit from TST to receive it.

UROLOGIC CLINICS OF NORTH AMERICA

THE CLINICS ARE AVAILABLE ONLINE!
Access your subscription at:
www.theclinics.com

Foreword
Hypogonadism

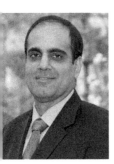

Samir S. Taneja, MD
Consulting Editor

My interest in Urology was originally sparked by the relationship of testosterone to prostate cancer. As a medical student interested in everything and nothing, I met a urologist by the name of Jack Grayhack and a scientist by the name of Chung Lee. Both had collaborated for years in the lab in trying to understand better what made prostate cells grow, become malignant, and proliferate. In learning about prostate cancer, I found it fascinating that a hormone important for essential bodily functions could be transformed into a driver of mortality—that changes in our cells could turn friend into foe. I wanted to understand this more, so I joined the lab, and my career in Urology began. The passion to understand this relationship, for me, has remained 28 years later.

In the field of prostate cancer, we have come full circle in regard to our perception of the importance of testosterone in prostate cancer. Since the description of the hormonal responsiveness of prostate cancer by Huggins in the 1960s, we went from believing castration was important for all, to believing it was beneficial only for some, to believing it was harmful to some, and now believing it may be harmful to many. We went from believing testosterone was bad, to now believing it is not only good but also essential for protection of the aging male.

It is now known that testosterone not only is an important factor in influencing prostate development, carcinogenesis, and cancer progression but also influences a variety of bodily functions, beyond the genitourinary tract. As men realize the benefits of testosterone replacement for decreased libido and reduced energy, and its use becomes more widespread, we have begun to ask about the risks.

Can it be safe for everyone? Can it be safe in every clinical scenario?

In the evolution of contemporary health care, integrated care models, linked to common disease states, will become a central point of access to the health care system. For men, the concerns about hypogonadism may serve as an inlet to evaluation for cardiac, metabolic, musculoskeletal, and malignant disease processes. As such, it is essential that urologists remain the most knowledgeable caregivers in regard to the state of hypogonadism, and, in doing so, become the gatekeepers in Men's Health. For that reason, this issue of *Urologic Clinics*, devoted to the hypogonadal male, carries great significance to me and is one I believe we should all read with focus. Our guest editor, my colleague and friend, Dr Joseph P. Alukal, has constructed a fantastic spectrum of articles related to every aspect of testosterone's relationship with bodily functions and disease processes to be considered in the aging male. As always, I am deeply indebted to Dr Alukal and all of the many outstanding authors who have graciously contributed to the issue. I think this one is a must-read for all urologists.

Samir S. Taneja, MD
Division of Urologic Oncology
Smilow Comprehensive Prostate Cancer Center
Department of Urology
NYU Langone Medical Center
150 East 32nd Street, Suite 200
New York, NY 10016, USA

E-mail address:
samir.taneja@nyumc.org

Urol Clin N Am 43 (2016) xv
http://dx.doi.org/10.1016/j.ucl.2016.03.002
0094-0143/16/$ – see front matter © 2016 Published by Elsevier Inc.

Preface
Hypogonadism

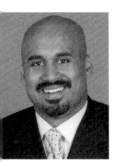

Joseph P. Alukal, MD
Editor

Hypogonadism (testosterone deficiency) is a prevalent condition that has become increasingly controversial. Recent studies raise the question of whether or not testosterone replacement is overprescribed and unacceptably risky from a cardiac health standpoint. This perception of risk is now present within the lay press and much of the lay population.

This controversy ignores the fact that hormone replacement therapy in male patients has been used for many years, and it has been studied from a number of different angles. The relationship between testosterone and prostate cancer physiology resulted in a Nobel Prize almost five decades ago; scientists have been studying testosterone and its relationship to sexual function, heart health, diabetes, bone density, and muscle development for more than one hundred years. Included in this issue is the clinical experience and research expertise of many of the leaders in this effort.

This issue of *Urologic Clinics of North America* is designed to help patients and practitioners better understand this common and controversial problem. A thorough discussion of the physiology of testosterone in the male, the options for testosterone replacement and their risks, as well as future directions for this field are included herein. Given the public health impact of this bothersome condition, this work is timely and needed; we hope it will guide clinicians in the proper management of their hypogonadal patients.

Joseph P. Alukal, MD
Male Reproductive Health
Departments of Urology, Obstetrics/Gynecology
New York University School of Medicine
150 East 32nd Street, 2nd Floor
New York, NY 10016, USA

E-mail address:
alukal@gmail.com

Urol Clin N Am 43 (2016) xvii
http://dx.doi.org/10.1016/j.ucl.2016.03.001
0094-0143/16/$ – see front matter © 2016 Published by Elsevier Inc.

urologic.theclinics.com

Physiology of the Hypothalamic Pituitary Gonadal Axis in the Male

Patricia Freitas Corradi, MD[a], Renato B. Corradi, MD[b],
Loren Wissner Greene, MD, MA[c],*

KEYWORDS

- Testosterone • Gonadotropin • Hypogonadism • Primary hypogonadism
- Secondary hypogonadism • Hypogonadotropic hypogonadism

KEY POINTS

- Testosterone synthesis and male fertility are controlled by a negative feedback mechanism between the hypothalamus, the pituitary, and the testis.
- Congenital or acquired conditions leading to a failure of hormone synthesis or action at any level of the hypothalamic-pituitary-gonadal axis result in the clinical syndrome of hypogonadism.
- Medications and contemporary diseases are major causes of impairment of male reproductive function. Novel therapies may improve spermatogenesis along with elevating testosterone levels in men.

INTRODUCTION

Reproductive function changes markedly during life in humans. Impeccable coordination of the hypothalamic-pituitary-gonadal axis is required for normal testicular function in the male, including normal testosterone production and male fertility. Pulsatile secretion of gonadotropin-releasing hormone (GnRH) by the hypothalamus stimulates the biosynthesis of pituitary gonadotropins, luteinizing hormone (LH), and follicle-stimulating hormone (FSH) that, in turn, sustain intragonadal testosterone production and spermatogenesis. A negative feedback mechanism, controlled by sufficient levels of testosterone, is responsible for decreasing both hypothalamic GnRH secretion into the portal circulation and gonadotropin release from the pituitary into the bloodstream.

Congenital or acquired conditions leading to a failure of hormone synthesis or action at any level of the axis result in the clinical syndrome of hypogonadism. Hypogonadism may be caused either by a primary testicular disease or by a secondary (or central) cause (eg, a hypothalamic or pituitary disorder). In the setting of acquired hypogonadism, comorbidities and use of medications are common causes of low testosterone and must be ruled out before making the diagnosis.

Despite the cause, end organ replacement therapy with natural testosterone is recommended for chronic use but with the understood general caveat that this treatment does not improve fertility. If medications that stimulate hypothalamic or pituitary function are successful, these agents may be used for several-month intervals to enhance spermatogenesis; however, their long-term use needs further investigation. In addition, novel therapeutic agents have been proposed to stimulate both testosterone and spermatogenesis. The understanding of hypothalamic-pituitary-gonadal axis physiology is the first step for the correct diagnosis

[a] Division of Endocrinology, New York University School of Medicine, 650 First Avenue, 7th Floor, New York, NY 10016, USA; [b] Urology Service, Department of Surgery, Memorial Sloan Kettering Cancer Center, 417 E 68th Street, New York, NY 10065, USA; [c] Bioethics and Medical Ethics, New York University School of Medicine, 650 First Avenue, 7th Floor, New York, NY 10016, USA
* Corresponding author.
E-mail address: loren.greene@nyumc.org

Urol Clin N Am 43 (2016) 151–162
http://dx.doi.org/10.1016/j.ucl.2016.01.001

and treatment of hypogonadism, a frequent condition affecting quality of life and causing other comorbidities including osteoporosis in men.

This article reviews the physiology of the brain-hypothalamic-pituitary-gonadal axis, to correlate it to disorders that can induce male hypogonadism, and discusses available and potential future treatment modalities.

ANATOMIC OVERVIEW OF THE HYPOTHALAMUS AND PITUITARY

The hypothalamus lies at the base of the brain, below the thalamus and the third ventricle, just above the optic chiasm and pituitary gland. It synthesizes and secretes certain neurohormones, often called *releasing hormones* or *hypothalamic hormones*, and these in turn stimulate or inhibit the secretion of pituitary hormones. The neurovascular link between hypothalamus and pituitary gland is the pituitary stalk, which comprises mainly neural and vascular components.

The pituitary gland, also known as the *hypophysis*, is located immediately beneath the hypothalamus, resting in a depression of the base of the skull called the *sella turcica* (Turkish saddle). The pituitary gland is entirely ectodermal in origin but is composed of 2 functionally distinct structures that differ in embryologic development and anatomy: the adenohypophysis (anterior pituitary) and the neurohypophysis (posterior pituitary). The adenohypophysis develops from an upward invagination of oral ectoderm named *Rathke's pouch*, whereas the neurohypophysis derives from a downward extension of neural ectoderm, the infundibulum.[1] Because the pituitary is just below the crossing of the visual nerves at the optic chiasm, pituitary tumors enlarging superiorly may affect superior temporal vision selectively.

The adenohypophysis is the manufacturer of an array of peptide hormones—gonadotropins (FSH and LH), adrenocorticotropin, growth hormone, prolactin, and thyroid-stimulating hormone (TSH)—and makes up roughly 80% of the pituitary gland. The release of these pituitary hormones is mediated by hypothalamic neurohormones that reach the adenohypophysis via a portal venous system.

Unlike the adenohypophysis, the neurohypophysis is not glandular and does not synthesize hormones. It stores and releases oxytocin and vasopressin, which are synthesized by neurosecretory cells of the hypothalamus. The neurohypophysis comprises axons of hypothalamic neurons; the neurohypophysis is, therefore, considered an extension of the hypothalamus.

CONTROL OF HYPOTHALAMIC SECRETION

In recent years, kisspeptin, a 54-amino-acid peptide, encoded by the KiSS-1 gene, was identified. Kisspeptin activates the G protein–coupled receptor (GPR54) of the hypothalamus. During pregnancy, kisspeptin levels increase 7000 times. Human placenta secretes varying lengths of the peptide, but the C-terminal 10-amino-acid portion is sufficient to activate GnRH receptors in the fetus, initiating function of the hypothalamic-pituitary-gonadal axis. Kisspeptin also provides the major trigger for puberty. In rat studies, chronic infusion of kisspeptin triggers precocious puberty and enables pubertal development in undernourished animals.[2]

NORMAL HYPOTHALAMIC REGULATION OF GONADOTROPINS

Secretion of pituitary gonadotropic hormones is regulated by the hypothalamic decapeptide hormone, GnRH, which binds to a membrane receptor on pituitary gonadotrophs, stimulating synthesis and secretion of both FSH and LH, the 2 pituitary gonadotropic hormones (**Fig. 1**).

Animal studies found that, in GnRH-deficient mice, pretreatment with GnRH led to both an increase in the gonadotropin content of the pituitary gland and[3] an induction of the expression of pituitary GnRH receptors.[4] Under certain physiologic conditions, GnRH receptor number varies and usually directly correlates with the gonadotropin secretory capacity of pituitary gonadotrophs.

Besides the number of GnRH receptors, pulsatile regimens of GnRH are required for the precision of pituitary gonadotropin signaling.[5] GnRH pulsatility seems to be an intrinsic function of hypothalamic cells, dependent on calcium, with communication similar to nerve synapse conduction.[6] Studies find a sequential response of gonadotropin secretion after exogenous GnRH administration in GnRH-deficient mice; there is an immediate and persistent increase in plasma FSH concentrations during the period of GnRH injections, whereas LH secretion requires a more prolonged and pulsatile GnRH therapy before LH is detected in the circulation.[7] Furthermore, these important data indicate that FSH continues to be synthesized and stored even in the absence of sustained GnRH administration, but continued GnRH stimulation is required for LH synthesis.

FOLLICLE-STIMULATING HORMONE, LUTEINIZING HORMONE, AND TESTICULAR FUNCTION

FSH and LH are heterodimers with structural similarities; each consists of α and β peptide

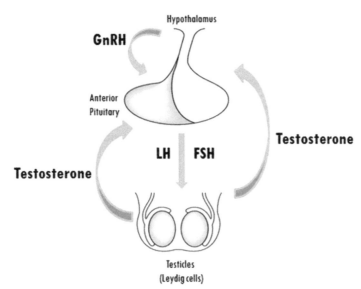

Fig. 1. Hypothalamic-pituitary-gonadal axis.

chain subunits, produced in the pituitary of both men and women. The α subunit is identical in both hormones; the β subunit, therefore, provides structural and biochemical specificity for receptor interactions and also determines the biologic specificity of the hormone. To date, hypogonadotropic hypogonadism (HH) owing to selective mutations in the FSH β or LH β subunit genes is rarely reported.[8]

FSH is required for the determination of the testicular Sertoli cell number and for induction and maintenance of spermatogenesis. In testes with a sufficient level of testosterone,[6] LH stimulates the secretion of gonadal steroids through Leydig cell activity. The same LH molecule stimulates estradiol synthesis in the ovary in women.[9] By activating the FSH receptor, FSH has specific function within the Sertoli cells of the testis, resulting in an increase in cyclic adenosine monophosphate, thereby activating a cyclic adenosine monophosphate–dependent protein kinase. This increase, in turn, increases protein synthesis of androgen-binding protein (sex hormone–binding globulin [SHBG]) and the aromatase enzyme CYP19, which converts testosterone to estradiol.[10]

Steroidogenesis, under the influence of LH acting through specific receptors found on the surface of the testicular Leydig cells, stimulates enzymatic conversion of precursor cholesterol into testosterone. Leydig cell secretion creates a high local concentration of testosterone in the testis; testosterone is also secreted into the circulation, with circulating testosterone levels occurring in a steep downhill concentration gradient from the testes, producing characteristic androgenic

effects on distant androgen-sensitive target tissues.[11] When testosterone levels are sufficient, the pituitary gland decreases the production and release of LH via a negative feedback mechanism, which also decreases GnRH and LH, thereby, decreasing testosterone levels. Apparently, much of the negative feedback regarding FSH occurs via the gonadal peptide hormones, inhibins, and activins, members of the transforming growth factor–β super family of molecules. Sertoli cells of the adult testes secrete both inhibins A and B, but the more important hormone is inhibin B, which suppresses FSH secretion, modulating the FSH stimulation by activins. Follistatins, produced within the pituitary, bind activins and further decrease their function. Beyond their negative pituitary feedback, inhibins function also throughout the reproductive hormonal axis and act locally as paracrine hormones within the testes.[12]

PERIPHERAL METABOLISM OF TESTOSTERONE

The testis contributes more than 95% of total circulating testosterone in the postpubertal man (the adrenal contributes the remainder). Testosterone is secreted into the circulation down a concentration gradient, where it equilibrates between protein-bound (98%) and free hormone (2%) fractions. Protein-bound testosterone binds either to low-affinity, high-availability proteins (primarily albumin) or to the high-affinity, low-abundance SHBG, a glycoprotein. The free hormone fraction is generally believed to be the biologically active form of testosterone. Once released in the bloodstream, testosterone reaches its peripheral sites of action, where it undergoes reversible and irreversible metabolism to other steroids with different activities (**Fig. 2**).

Although only approximately 5% of serum testosterone produced in men undergoes 5α-reduction to dihydrotestosterone (DHT), many of the important functions of testosterone are mediated by this potent metabolite.[13] Testosterone and DHT bind to a common androgen receptor; however, DHT has 2 to 3 times greater androgen receptor affinity than testosterone; moreover, the dissociation rate of testosterone from the androgen receptor is 5-fold faster than DHT.[14] Also, DHT cannot be aromatized to estrogen. During embryogenesis, DHT has an essential role in the formation of the male external genitalia, whereas in the adult, DHT acts as the primary androgen in the prostate and in hair follicles.[15] If there is insufficient conversion of testosterone to DHT, owing to deficient 5α-reductase enzyme, as in the genetic "penis at 14" syndrome (5α-reductase deficiency), the infant male will have a feminine appearance with small phallus and internal testes. However, after puberty, the penis enlarges and the male appearance ensues under the influence of mature testosterone levels.[16] Interestingly, this gender transformation is completely accepted socially and psychologically in certain inbred communities of the Dominican Republic and Greece, and the adult male has normal reproductive function. (As a matter of fact, this issue is accurately addressed in the Pulitzer Prize-winning novel Middlesex, by Jeffrey Eugenides published in 2002.)

In the adult, as testosterone is converted to DHT, the prostate gland grows and male pattern hair loss proceeds. Understanding this biology, drug blockade with a 5α-reductase antagonist like finasteride may be used to decrease prostate size in benign prostatic hypertrophy and to slow male pattern balding.[17] This drug is dangerous for a pregnant woman to use, as it would also impair the development of a phallus in the male fetus, similar to the block in the previously mentioned "penis at 14" syndrome.

In peripheral tissues, testosterone can also be converted to estrogens through the action of microsomal P450 enzyme CYP19 aromatase, expressed in many sites, including placenta, gonads, brain, and fat. More than 80% of circulating estradiol in men is derived from the aromatization of testosterone[18]; thus, male hypogonadism leads to a consequent hypoestrogenism. In men with deficient aromatization of testosterone to estrogen, there are high levels of testosterone, yet decreased levels of estrogen lead to increased levels of LH, a demonstration that lack of estrogen feedback to the pituitary is more important than feedback from testosterone.[19] Together with evidence of the important role of estrogen in bone metabolism, Finkelstein and colleagues[20] found

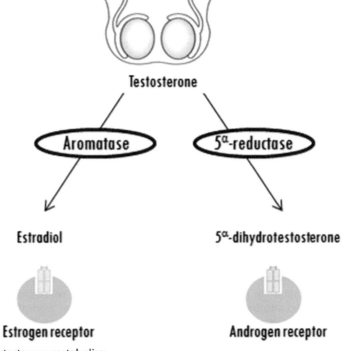

Fig. 2. Peripheral testosterone metabolism.

that estrogens also play a fundamental role in the regulation of body fat and sexual function in men. On the other hand, in situations of fat accumulation, such as obesity or insulin resistance, the increased adiposity is associated with increased aromatase conversion of testosterone to estrogens in fat tissue, often resulting in gynecomastia, sometimes with lower levels of testosterone.

SEXUAL DEVELOPMENT IN MALES

Pulsatile secretion of GnRH from the hypothalamus is required for the maintenance of reproductive function; however, the pattern of GnRH-induced gonadotropin secretion is constantly changing during sexual development. Neuroendocrine stimulation of the reproductive axis is initiated during fetal development. Although GnRH neurons are seen earlier in fetal life, the connection between these neurons and the portal system of the hypothalamus and pituitary becomes functional around 16 weeks of gestation.[21] Hypothalamic GnRH neurons are functional at birth but, after the perinatal androgen surge, remain tonically suppressed during infantile life. During childhood, the hypothalamic-pituitary axis is characterized by low pulse frequency and low amplitude GnRH secretion.

The precise neuroendocrine trigger of puberty is not fully understood. Nevertheless, its onset is marked by sleep-entrained reactivation of the reproductive axis characterized by a remarkable increase in the amplitude of LH pulses with a lesser change in frequency. Initially, the nighttime elevation of LH secretion stimulates gonadal secretion of sex steroids, which return to prepubertal levels during the daytime. As puberty progresses, gonadotropins are secreted during both day and night, allowing sexual development to be completed.[22] The testicular output of testosterone gains control over the hypothalamic discharge of GnRH, maintaining a constant frequency of LH pulses, and the sleep-entrained differences in testosterone and LH become negligible. By this time, the increased level of testosterone, along with its conversion to the active metabolite DHT, causes deepening of the voice, secondary sex hair distribution, enlargement of testicles, growth of the penis, and increased libido. Higher levels of testosterone itself, and by its conversion to estrogen, lead to development of muscle mass, bone maturation, and accelerated bone growth until closure of the epiphyses of long bones.

During adulthood, pulsatile GnRH continues to stimulate biosynthesis of LH and FSH that, in turn, sustain intragonadal testosterone production and spermatogenesis as well as systemic testosterone secretion and virilization.

HYPOGONADOTROPIC HYPOGONADISM

Failure of the episodic GnRH secretion or action, or disruption of gonadotropin secretion, results in the clinical syndrome of HH. This condition can be caused by either pituitary or hypothalamic disorders and is referred to as *secondary* or *tertiary* hypogonadism, respectively. Secondary and tertiary HH can be distinguished from primary or testicular causes by the demonstration of low/normal gonadotropin levels in the setting of low testosterone concentration (**Table 1**).

A high number of loci are associated with congenital GnRH deficiency and mutations in the GnRH receptor in the pituitary. The mutated GPR54 receptor, not receptive to kisspeptin stimulation, may cause HH in humans.[2]

Although rare, congenital abnormalities are well understood and described causes of deficient GnRH secretion and can occur either in isolation (normosmic congenital HH) or in association with anosmia or hyposmia, which is named *Kallmann syndrome* (KS). To define the genetic and phenotypic variability of GnRH deficiency syndrome in humans, a detailed family history of 106 GnRH-deficient patients collected by Waldstreicher and colleagues[23] found an equal occurrence of KS and idiopathic HH. Their observations in this cohort of patients found the predominance of males (85 males vs 21 females) and the autosomal transmission in familial cases. Despite prior studies suggesting an X-linked form of KS, in this series, this finding was not consistent. Therefore, they concluded that most often, this abnormality occurred sporadically, and many were novel autosomal mutations.

On immunoreactive labeling, normal and KS human nasal epithelium obtained from aborted human fetuses contains both sex steroid (estrogen and progesterone) and GnRH receptors. Because the olfactory neurons and GnRH neurons have a common embryologic origin, the congruence of GnRH deficiency and anosmia as related abnormalities of neuronal migration from the cribriform plate through the olfactory bulb and tract to the hypothalamus during organogenesis is not surprising. One of the mutations identified in X-linked KS is in the *KAL1* gene, encoding anosmin-1, a neural cell adhesion glycoprotein critical to growth and movement of the GnRH neurons.[24] Abnormalities affecting p*KAL*, the promoter region of this gene, have also been found. Absent olfactory tracts may be found on brain MRI (see **Fig. 4**).[25] The interconnected nature of smell and sex hormone control

Table 1
Causes of hypogonadism in males

Primary (Increased LH/FSH, Low T)		Secondary (Normal/Low LH/FSH, Low T)	
Congenital	Acquired	Congenital	Acquired
Klinefelter syndrome	Chronic renal failure	KS	Hyperprolactinemia
Androgen synthesis disorder	Hepatic cirrhosis	DAX-1 mutation	Critical illness
Mutation of FSH receptor gene	Hemochromatosis	GPR-54 mutation	Chronic systemic illness
Cryptorchidism	Human immunodeficiency virus/AIDS	Leptin or leptin receptor mutation	Diabetes mellitus
Undescended testicles	Infections (eg, mumps orchitis)	Prader-Willi syndrome	Obesity
Varicocele	Radiation	Gonadotropin subunit mutation	Neoplasms
Myotonic dystrophy	Trauma		Infiltrative diseases (eg, sarcoidosis, histiocytosis, tuberculosis)
	Toxins (eg, ethanol)		Pituitary apoplexy
	Autoimmune damage		Pituitary trauma
	Drugs		Ethanol
			Drugs

Abbreviation: T, testosterone.

was shown by demonstration that human fetal olfactory reception provokes GnRH gene expression with GnRH protein secretion (Even later, in adult mammals, the sense of smell, transmitted by pheromones, may lead to perception of ovulatory status and elicit reproductive behaviors).[26] Along with low testosterone, decreased fertility, and anosmia, KS individuals may have other neurologic changes and cardiac conditions.

Rare mutations of the LH-β or FSH-β subunits cause resistant syndromes. Acquired causes of HH are far more common and may be caused by any disorder that affects the hypothalamus itself. In adults, HH can be induced by emotional stress, physical exercise, anorexia, sleep deprivation, alcohol, and medications (**Box 1**). The hypothalamus, in turn, is controlled by brain centers responding to stimulation from the environment affecting mood and status. For example, recent studies found that fatherhood may lower testosterone levels,[27] whereas situations in which an individual is angry or exerts power might increase testosterone levels.[28]

Aging, obesity, and type 2 diabetes are known risk factors for hypogonadism in men. Studies have found that testosterone production slowly and continuously decreases as a result of aging, although the rate of decline varies, unlike women, who experience a rapid decline in sex hormone levels during menopause. Both cross-sectional and longitudinal studies found a decline in serum testosterone concentration, an increase in SHBG concentration, and a decrease in free testosterone with age. Also, a significant percentage of men older than 60 years have serum testosterone levels that are less than the lower limits of young adult (age 20–30 years) men.

Similar to the projections for an aging population, an increased incidence of secondary hypogonadism can be a result of the increasing incidence of obesity. The proposed causes for the effects of obesity on testosterone levels include increased clearance or aromatization of testosterone into estrogen in the adipose tissue (see **Fig. 2**) and increased formation of inflammatory cytokines, which hinder the secretion of the GnRH.[29] Another common cause of hypogonadism, diabetes mellitus, was found to be associated with primary testicular failure and low testosterone levels and also may produce HH with low pituitary gonadotropin levels.[30]

Some drugs, including synthetic anabolic steroids and other corticosteroids, may result in hypogonadism with decreased endogenous male hormone production and reproductive failure. The negative hypothalamic-pituitary feedback from exogenous androgens causes a functional form of HH, and the decreased gonadotropin secretion, in turn, lowers both endogenous testosterone and DHT secretion and impairs spermatogenesis, shrinking testicular volume and decreasing fertility.[31] Simultaneously, well-described side effects include loss of libido, erectile dysfunction, gynecomastia, increased acne, profuse sweating, and increased prostate size.

The effects might be the same if an exogenous testosterone product (intramuscular or transdermal) is used. If a 5α-reductase inhibitor is used at the same time as the androgen, male pattern hair loss does not proceed. In addition, testosterone alone or testosterone administered in combination with the 5α-reductase inhibitor, finasteride, is associated with similar increase in hematocrit and incidence of polycythemia.[32] A thorough medical history in the hypogonadal man should include the use of exogenous synthetic or natural androgens.

ANDROGEN INSENSITIVITY SYNDROME

Androgen insensitivity syndrome is the largest single entity that leads to male undermasculinization.[33] Androgen insensitivity syndrome can be defined as an X-linked disorder caused by mutations in the androgen receptor gene that lead to complete or partial resistance to the biological actions of androgens in an XY boy or man with normal testis determination and production of age-appropriate androgen concentrations.

In the complete form of androgen insensitivity, the phenotype is a complete feminization of an XY individual. Androgen insensitivity is often diagnosed by chance, during the investigation of primary amenorrhea in adolescence, or inguinal swellings in an infant. The presence of undescended tests is associated with abnormal

---

Box 1
Medications that could potentially cause hypogonadism

Glucocorticoids

Ketoconazole

Chemotherapeutic drugs (eg, alkylating agents)

Opiates

GnRH analogues

Anabolic steroids

Metoclopramide

Spironolactone

testicular development and an increased risk of germ cell malignancy.[34] When complete androgen insensitivity is diagnosed in infancy, early gonadectomy with puberty induction can be done later, or gonadectomy can be delayed until early adulthood, as clinical studies find that the risk of premalignant change in germ cells is low before and during puberty.[35] Hence, feminizing hormone therapy is required to induce or maintain secondary sexual characteristics. Estrogen is also important to optimize bone mass accrual.[36]

The clinical presentation of partial androgen insensitivity syndrome varies according to the degree of responsiveness of the external genitalia to androgens. Therefore, the determination of gender to be raised is usually determined by the dominant phenotype.

Androgen insensitivity presents with an endocrine profile of a hormone-resistant state: testosterone levels are either within or greater than the normal range for men and boys, and LH concentrations are inappropriately increased. Concentrations of FSH and inhibin are generally normal. Serum anti-Müllerian hormone measurement suggests the presence of testes.[37]

ABNORMALITIES IN TESTICULAR FUNCTION

The control of gonadotropin production, with negative feedback, can be seen in Klinefelter syndrome. Klinefelter syndrome is characterized by the presence of one or more extra X chromosomes, and the karyotype 47 XXY or variants XXY/XY or XXXY. It is the most common chromosomal abnormality with a prevalence of 1:600 in males in some series; Klinefelter syndrome is the most common genetic cause of small testis and azoospermia.[38] The testicular histology of Klinefelter patients is somewhat variable but often includes progressive hyalinization of the seminiferous tubules with age-related loss of germ cells,[39] with Leydig-cell hyperplasia yet inefficient androgen production by Leydig cells.[40] Because of this extensive testicular involvement, gonadotropin levels increase, the LH responding to the low level of negative feedback from testosterone. At the same time, perhaps in response to abnormal spermatogenesis, FSH secretion is stimulated, resulting in high plasma levels of FSH.

In several described cases, testosterone synthesis is impaired owing to abnormalities of the LH receptor gene, leading to LH resistance in the testes with Leydig cell hypoplasia. Affected XY patients present with variable fetal development of masculine features (ie, micropenis, feminized external genitalia) and primary hypogonadism. In this condition, the LH level is high, although testosterone level remains low in the plasma.[41]

Cancer treatment also has influence on the male reproductive system. Some chemotherapeutic agents and radiation therapy can induce infertility by damaging the seminiferous tubules and by damaging spermatogonia.[42] Concomitant weight loss may further damage the hypothalamic-pituitary-testicular axis.

DIAGNOSIS

Gonadal steroids regulate pituitary gonadotropin secretion in part by altering the amplitude or frequency of hypothalamic GnRH release.[5] The presence of such a negative feedback control by the testis on pituitary FSH and LH secretion is best shown by the rapid increase of FSH and LH after castration. Given its short half-life, in the adult male, LH is secreted in pulses approximately every 2 hours.[43] However, considerable variability is observed in LH pulse patterns, and there is a wide range of testosterone secretory patterns. Comorbidities, infections, and concomitant use of drugs that could alter hormonal synthesis or secretion at any axis level must be ruled out. Also, within-patient variation must be considered when interpreting single LH and testosterone measurements obtained during the evaluation of a male with suspected hypogonadism. Young men exhibit a diurnal variation, with highest values of testosterone at about 8 AM and lowest about 8 PM, but older men have little variation.[44] Sometimes men who are found initially to have a low testosterone concentration will have a normal level on repeat early morning testing.[45]

The diagnosis of androgen deficiency should be made only in men with consistent symptoms and signs (**Box 2**) and unequivocally low early-morning serum testosterone levels that are less than the lower limit of the normal range (usually <300 ng/dL)[46] in at least 2 different morning measurements. Free or bioavailable testosterone levels may be useful in men with suspected SHBG abnormalities caused by aging, obesity, chronic illness, thyroid disease, or liver disease.[47] Gonadotropins should be measured to elucidate the integrity of the central portion of reproductive axis. Additional pituitary hormone testing, such as an elevation of prolactin, may be useful to confirm a diagnosis of secondary hypogonadism with pituitary disease. In HH, stimulation with GnRH (also called LHRH) infusion to see pituitary gonadotropin (LH and FSH) response is useful to separate hypothalamic causes that do respond from the nonresponsive pituitary causes.[48] Karyotyping should be used to exclude Klinefelter

Box 2
Signs and symptoms of hypogonadism in the adult male

Sexual dysfunction: reduced libido, diminished penile sensation, erectile dysfunction, difficulty attaining orgasm, reduced ejaculate, oligospermia

Regression of secondary sexual characteristics

Reduced bone mass or bone mineral density

Muscle wasting

Gynecomastia

Reduced energy, fatigue

Anemia

Increased abdominal adiposity

Depressed mood

Difficulty concentrating

Changes in cholesterol levels

syndrome in the suspected individual (**Fig. 3**). Pituitary MRI may find pituitary and hypothalamic disease and even show the absence of olfactory structures in KS (**Fig. 4**).[24]

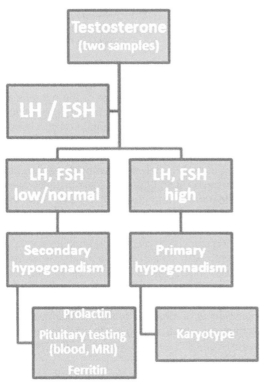

Fig. 3. Algorithm for clinical diagnosis of hypogonadism.

TREATMENT

Once hypogonadism is diagnosed, chronic hormone replacement is the preferable therapy using testosterone preparations. Nevertheless, because exogenous testosterone formulations cannot mimic the natural endogenous pathway of hypothalamus-pituitary hormonal axis, suppression of the hypothalamic-pituitary-gonadal axis is inevitable via a negative feedback mechanism. Low levels of GnRH, in turn, further decrease production of LH and FSH by the pituitary gland. The low LH levels translate to low testosterone production by the Leydig cells in the testis.

If prolactin is elevated, dopaminergic drugs including bromocriptine or cabergoline may be used to suppress prolactin and often enhance gonadotropin secretion.

LH and human chorionic gonadotropin (hCG) are heterodimeric glycoproteins that share a common α subunit. The rate-limiting step in LH and hCG production is the transcription of the β subunit. They have different stability, circulating half-life, and affinity to receptor; however, as a result of minimal structural differences, they both bind and activate a common receptor in the gonads. Although each hormone triggers a particular cascade of events after receptor binding,[49] pharmacologic hCG functions as an LH analogue and is known to stimulate testosterone synthesis in Leydig cells.[50]

In patients who have undergone hypophysectomy, or in other pituitary diseases, often hCG alone can sustain spermatogenesis.[51] Men must continue subcutaneous or intramuscular injections of hCG, 1500 to 2000 IU 3 times a week for at least 6 months, as sperm production takes several months. After several months of hCG alone, if adequate spermatogenesis has not occurred, human menopausal gonadotropins or recombinant FSH can be added as an effective regimen in inducing spermatogenesis in male patients with idiopathic HH. However, there is insufficient information about the therapeutic or adverse effects of chronic hCG or recombinant FSH treatment of hypogonadism.

With hypothalamic disease, pulsatile subcutaneous or intravenous GnRH, delivered with an infusion pump and tubing (similar to an insulin pump), may be used to stimulate appropriate pituitary gonadotropin secretion. Obviously, this approach would not work in pituitary disease, and, like pituitary disease, would require months of therapy.

NOVEL THERAPEUTICS

Studies on estrogen feedback on the hypothalamic-pituitary axis in the human have

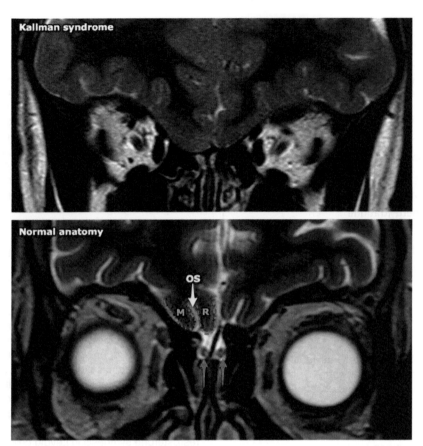

Fig. 4. The normal anatomy consists of the olfactory bulbs (*blue arrows*) located in the olfactory grooves of the anterior cranial fossa. The inferior surface of the frontal lobes usually consists gyrus rectus (R) separated from the medial orbital gyrus (M) by the olfactory sulcus (*yellow arrow*). These are absent in KS. (*Courtesy of* Dr Frank Gaillard, Radiopaedia.org, Melbourne, Australia. rID: 6083.)

found that estrogen inhibits LH secretion by decreasing LH pulse amplitude and LH responsiveness to GnRH. Also, the use of aromatase inhibitors—a class of medication that functions to block the conversion of androgens to estrogens—was found to increase LH pulse frequency,[52] whereas testosterone level remains high. In addition, the increased gonadotropins further stimulate endogenous testosterone production, stimulate spermatogenesis, and improve male fertility. However there are risks in the chronic use of these medications, including bone loss, as most of the effect of testosterone on bone is mediated through estrogen.

Because hypogonadism is often associated with changes in the testosterone/estrogen ratio owing to increased levels of estrogens,[53] a different class of antiestrogens could also be used. Clomiphene citrate is a weak estrogen receptor antagonist and, thus, may be considered a selective estrogen receptor modulator. Clomiphene citrate competes with estradiol for the

estrogen receptors at the level of the hypothalamus and blocks the normal negative feedback mechanism of circulating estradiol on the hypothalamus, preventing estrogen from limiting the production of GnRH. The resulting increased amount of GnRH stimulates the pituitary gland to release more LH and FSH, resulting in an increase in testosterone and sperm production by the testis.[54] As sperm production proceeds over several months, a short course of clomiphene may increase sperm production enough to obtain sufficient sperm to achieve pregnancy. However, more prolonged use of clomiphene in men has not been studied sufficiently to recommend its chronic use to increase testosterone and spermatogenesis. In phase III trials, a similar drug, enclomiphene citrate, was found to similarly improve testosterone and spermatogenesis simultaneously in HH.[55]

In Klinefelter syndrome, isolated rests of areas with spermatogenesis have been successfully aspirated from the testes, especially in younger men.[56] Even a few healthy sperm might be enough to achieve fertilization, through techniques such as ICSI (intracytoplasmic sperm insemination) in which a sperm is injected directly into an ovum obtained through in vitro fertilization.

SUMMARY

Testosterone synthesis and male fertility are the results of the perfect coordination of the hypothalamic-pituitary-gonadal axis. A negative feedback finely controls the secretion of hormones at the 3 levels. Congenital or acquired disturbance at any level leads to an impairment of reproductive function and the clinical syndrome of hypogonadism. In some cases, this condition is reversible. Once the diagnosis is made, testosterone replacement therapy is the standard therapy; however, novel therapies may improve spermatogenesis while elevating testosterone levels.

REFERENCES

1. Sheng HZ, Westphal H. Early steps in pituitary organogenesis. Trends Genet 1999;15(6):236–40.
2. Dhillo WS, Chaudhri OB, Patterson M. Kisspeptin-54 stimulates the hypothalamic-pituitary gonadal axis in human males. J Clin Endocrinol Metab 2005;90(12): 6609–61.
3. Young LS, Speight A, Charlton HM, et al. Pituitary gonadotropin-releasing hormone receptor regulation in the hypogonadotrophic hypogonadal (hpg) mouse. Endocrinology 1983;113(1):55–61.
4. Charlton HM, Halpin DM, Iddon C, et al. The effects of daily administration of single and multiple injections of gonadotropin-releasing hormone on pituitary and gonadal function in the hypogonadal (hpg) mouse. Endocrinology 1983;113(2):535–44.
5. Santen RJ, Bardin CW. Episodic luteinizing hormone secretion in man. Pulse analysis, clinical interpretation, physiologic mechanisms. J Clin Invest 1973; 52(10):2617–28.
6. Wetsel WC, Valença MM, Merchenthaler I, et al. Intrinsic pulsatile secretory activity of immortalized luteinizing hormone-releasing hormone-secreting neurons. Proc Natl Acad Sci U S A 1992;89:4149–53.
7. Marshall JC. Idiopathic hypogonadotropic hypogonadism in men: dependence of the hormone responses to gonadotropin- releasing hormone (GnRH) on the magnitude of the endogenous GnRH secretory defect. J Clin Endocrinol Metab 1985;61(6):1118–25.
8. Trarbach EB, Silveira LG, Latronico AC. Genetic insights into human isolated gonadotropin deficiency. Pituitary 2007;10(4):381–91.
9. O'Shaughnessy PJ, Monteiro A, Verhoeven G, et al. Effect of FSH on testicular morphology and spermatogenesis in gonadotrophin-deficient hypogonadal mice lacking androgen receptors. Reproduction 2010;139(1):177–84.
10. Means AR, Fakunding JL, Huckins C, et al. Follicle-stimulating hormone, the Sertoli cell, and spermatogenesis. Recent Prog Horm Res 1976;32:477.
11. Handelsman DJ. Testosterone: use, misuse and abuse. Med J Aust 2006;185(8):436–9.
12. Louise MB, Blount AL, Leal AMO, et al. Autocrine/paracrine regulation of pituitary function by activin, inhibin and follistatin. Mol Cell Endocrinol 2004;225:29–36.
13. Russel D, Wilson J. Steroid 5a reductase two genes/ two enzymes. Annu Rev Biochem 1994;63:25–61.
14. Grino PB, Griffin JE, Wilson JD. Testosterone at high concentrations interacts with the human androgen receptor similarly to dihydrotestosterone. Endocrinology 1990;126(2):1165–72.
15. Amory JK, Anawalt BD, Matsumoto AM, et al. The effect of 5alpha-reductase inhibition with dutasteride and finasteride on bone mineral density, serum lipoproteins, hemoglobin, prostate specific antigen and sexual function in healthy young men. J Urol 2008; 179(6):2333–8.
16. Kang HJ, Imperato-McGinley J, Zhu YS, et al. The effect of 5a-reductase-2 deficiency on human fertility. Fertil Sterility 2014;101(2):310–6.
17. Zhu Y-S, Imperato-McGinley JL. 5α-reductase isozymes and androgen actions in the prostate. Ann N Y Acad Sci 2009;1155(1):43–56.
18. Longcope C, Kato T, Horton R. Conversion of blood androgens to estrogens in normal adult men and women. J Clin Invest 1969;48(12):2191–201.
19. Leder BZ, LeBlanc KM, Schoenfeld DA, et al. Differential effects of androgens and estrogens on bone turnover in normal men. J Clin Endocrinol Metab 2003;88(1):204–10.
20. Finkelstein JS, Lee H, Burnett-Bowie S-AM, et al. Gonadal Steroids and Body Composition, Strength, and Sexual Function in Men. N Engl J Med 2013; 369(11):1011–22.
21. Waldhauser F, Weibenbacher G, Frisch H, et al. Pulsatile secretion of gonadotropins in early infancy. Eur J Pediatr 1981;137:71–4.
22. Boyar RM, Rosenfeld RS, Kapen S, et al. Human puberty. Simultaneous augmented secretion of luteinizing hormone and testosterone during sleep. J Clin Invest 1974;54(3):609–18.
23. Waldstreicher J, Seminara SB, Jameson L, et al. The genetic and clinical heterogeneity of gonadotropin-releasing hormone deficiency in the human. J Clin Endocrinol Metab 1996;81(12):4388–95.
24. Soussi-Yanicostas N, Faivre-Sarrailh C, Hardelin JP, et al. Anosmin-1 underlying the X chromosome-linked Kallmann syndrome is an adhesion molecule that can modulate neurite growth in a cell-type specific manner. J Cell Sci 1998;111:2953–65.
25. Quinton R, Duke VM, de Zoysa PA, et al. The neuroradiology of kallmann's syndrome: a genotypic and

phenotypic analysis. J Clin Endocrinol Metab 1996; 81:3010–7.

26. Barni T, Maggi M, Fantoni G, et al. Sex steroids and odorants modulate gonadotropin-releasing hormone secretion in primary cultures of human olfactory cells. J Clin Endocrinol Metab 1999;84(11):4266–73.

27. Harman SM, Metter EJ, Tobin JD, et al. Longitudinal effects of aging on serum total and free testosterone levels in healthy men. J Clin Endocrinol Metab 2014; 86(2):724–31.

28. Van Anders SM, Steiger J, Goldey KL. Effects of gendered behavior on testosterone in women and men. Proc Natl Acad Sci U S A 2015;112(45):13805–10.

29. Zumoff B, Strain GW, Miller LK, et al. Plasma free and non-sex-hormone-binding-globulin-bound testosterone are decreased in obese men in proportion to their degree of obesity. J Clin Endocrinol Metab 1990;71(4):929–31.

30. Dhindsa S, Prabhakar S, Sethi M, et al. Frequent Occurrence of Hypogonadotropic Hypogonadism in Type 2 Diabetes. J Clin Endocrinol Metab 2004; 89(11):5462–8.

31. Karila T, Hovatta O. Concomitant abuse of anabolic androgenic steroids and human chorionic gonadotrophin impairs spermatogenesis in power athletes. Int J Sports Med 2004;25(4):257–63.

32. Page ST, Amory JK, Bowman FD, et al. Exogenous testosterone (T) alone or with finasteride increases physical performance, grip strength, and lean body mass in older men with low serum T. J Clin Endocrinol Metab 2005;90(3):1502–10.

33. Ahmed SF, Cheng A, Hughes IA. Assessment of the gonadotrophin-gonadal axis in androgen insensitivity syndrome. Arch Dis Child 1999;80(4):324–9.

34. Manuel M, Katayama PK, Jones HW. The age of occurrence of gonadal tumors in intersex patients with a Y chromosome. Am J Obstet Gynecol 1976; 124(3):293–300.

35. Hannema SE, Scott IS, Rajpert-De Meyts E, et al. Testicular development in the complete androgen insensitivity syndrome. J Pathol 2006;208(4):518–27.

36. Bertelloni S, Dati E, Baroncelli GI, et al. Hormonal management of complete androgen insensitivity syndrome from adolescence onward. Horm Res Paediatr 2011;76(6):428–33.

37. Hughes IA, Davies JD, Bunch TI, et al. Androgen insensitivity syndrome. Lancet 2012;380(9851):1419–28.

38. Bojesen A, Gravholt CH. Klinefelter syndrome in clinical practice. Nat Clin Pract Urol 2007;4(4):192–204.

39. Muller J, Skakkebaek NE, Ratcliffe SG. Quantified testicular histology in boys with sex chromosome abnormalities. Int J Androl 1995;18(2):57–62.

40. Schirren C, Toyosi JO, Wurst I. Testicular histology in Klinefelter's syndrome. Int J Androl 1970;2(2):187–97.

41. Tsigos C, Latronico C, Chrousos GP. Luteinizing hormone resistance syndromes. Ann N Y Acad Sci 1997;816:263–73.

42. Howell SJ, Shalet SM. Spermatogenesis after cancer treatment: damage and recovery. J Natl Cancer Inst Monogr 2005;(34):12–7.

43. Spratt DI, O'Dea LS, Schoenfeld D, et al. Neuroendocrine-gonadal axis in men: frequent sampling of LH, FSH, and testosterone. Am J Physiol 1988;254: 58–66.

44. Bremner WJ, Vitiello MV, Prinz PN. Loss of circadian rhythmicity in blood testosterone levels with aging in normal men. J Clin Endocrinol Metab 1983;56(6): 1278–81.

45. Brambilla DJ, O'Donnell AB, Matsumoto AM, et al. Intraindividual variation in levels of serum testosterone and other reproductive and adrenal hormones in men. Clin Endocrinol (Oxf) 2007;67(6):853–62.

46. Basaria S. Male hypogonadism. Lancet 2014; 383(9924):1250–63.

47. Feldman HA, Longcope C, Derby CA, et al. Age trends in the level of serum testosterone and other hormones in middle-aged men: longitudinal results from the Massachusetts male aging study. J Clin Endocrinol Metab 2002;87(2):589–98.

48. Crowley WF Jr, Beitins IZ, Vale W, et al. The biologic activity of a potent analogue of gonadotropin-releasing hormone in normal and hypogonadotropic men. N Engl J Med 1980;302(19):1052–7.

49. Choi J, Smitz J. Luteinizing hormone and human chorionic gonadotropin: origins of difference. Mol Cell Endocrinol 2014;383(1–2):203–13.

50. Matsumoto AM. Testosterone administration in older men. Endocrinol Metab Clin North Am 2013;42(2): 271–86.

51. Zhang M, Tong G, Liu Y, et al. Sequential versus continual purified urinary FSH/hCG in men with idiopathic hypogonadotropic hypogonadism. J Clin Endocrinol Metab 2015;100(6):2449–55.

52. Hayes FJ, Seminara SB, Decruz S, et al. Aromatase inhibition in the human male reveals a hypothalamic site of estrogen feedback. J Clin Endocrinol Metab 2000;85(9):3027–35.

53. Tilbrook AJ, De Kretser DM, Cummins JT, et al. The negative feedback effects of testicular steroids are predominantly at the hypothalamus in the ram. Endocrinology 1991;129(6):3080–92.

54. Shabsigh A, Kang Y, Shabsign R, et al. Clomiphene citrate effects on testosterone/estrogen ratio in male hypogonadism. J Sex Med 2005;2(5):716–21.

55. Kim ED, McCullough A, Kaminetsky J. Oral enclomiphene citrate raises testosterone and preserves sperm counts in obese hypogonadal men, unlike topical testosterone: restoration instead of replacement. BJU Int 2015. [Epub ahead of print].

56. Bryson CF, Ramasamy R, Sheehan M, et al. Severe testicular atrophy does not affect the success of microdissection testicular sperm extraction. J Urol 2014; 191(1):175–8.

Hypogonadism
Its Prevalence and Diagnosis

Anna Ross, MD[a], Shalender Bhasin, MB, BS[b],*

KEYWORDS

- Hypogonadism • Prevalence • Diagnosis • Androgen deficiency

KEY POINTS

- It is important to distinguish organic hypogonadism due to known diseases of the testes, pituitary, and the hypothalamus for which testosterone therapy is indicated from the age-related decline in testosterone levels, in which neither the clinical benefits nor the long-term risks have been clearly demonstrated in randomized trials.
- The prevalence of organic hypogonadism due to known diseases of the testes, pituitary, and the hypothalamus is not known.
- The diagnosis of hypogonadism should be based on the ascertainment of signs and symptoms of androgen deficiency along with unequivocally low levels of circulating testosterone on at least 2 occasions, using a reliable assay.
- Measure free testosterone using an accurate method when alterations in binding protein concentrations are suspected.
- Primary hypogonadism can be distinguished from secondary hypogonadism by measurement of luteinizing hormone and follicle-stimulating hormone concentrations.

INTRODUCTION

Androgen deficiency syndromes in men result from diminished production of testosterone due to defects at one or more levels of the hypothalamic-pituitary-testicular axis. Testosterone is the most important androgen in men; more than 90% of circulating testosterone is derived from the Leydig cells under the influence of pulsatile gonadotropin-releasing hormone (GnRH) secretion from the hypothalamus and luteinizing hormone (LH) secretion from the pituitary. Although LH is the primary regulator of testicular testosterone production, follicle-stimulating hormone (FSH), in conjunction with high intratesticular testosterone concentrations, is essential for initiating and maintaining spermatogenesis. Circulating testosterone is bound largely to sex hormone–binding globulin (SHBG)

Disclosures: Dr A. Ross has no commercial or financial conflicts of interest to disclose. Dr S. Bhasin reports receiving grants from Abbvie Pharmaceuticals; research grants outside the submitted work from Regeneron Pharmaceuticals and Eli Lilly, which are administered by the Brigham and Women's Hospital; personal fees from Novartis, Sanofi, Eli Lilly & Co, and Abbvie. S. Bhasin has a financial interest in Function Promoting Therapies, LLC, a company aiming to develop innovative solutions that enhance precision and accuracy in clinical decision making and facilitate personalized therapeutic choices in reproductive health. S. Bhasin's interests were reviewed and are managed by Brigham and Women's Hospital and Partners HealthCare in accordance with their conflict of interest policies. He has served as the chair of the American Board of Internal Medicine Endocrinology Board Examination Writing Committee and as the chair of the Endocrine Society's expert panel that wrote the clinical guideline for testosterone therapy.
[a] Research Program in Men's Health: Aging and Metabolism, Brigham and Women's Hospital, 221 Longwood Avenue, Boston, MA 02115, USA; [b] Research Program in Men's Health: Aging and Metabolism, The Center for Clinical Investigation, Brigham and Women's Hospital, Harvard Medical School, 221 Longwood Avenue, Boston, MA 02115, USA
* Corresponding author.
E-mail address: sbhasin@partners.org

Urol Clin N Am 43 (2016) 163–176
http://dx.doi.org/10.1016/j.ucl.2016.01.002
0094-0143/16/$ – see front matter © 2016 Elsevier Inc. All rights reserved.

and to albumin, and to a much smaller extent to orosomucoid and cortisol-binding protein; only 1.0% to 4.0% is free.[1–5] Defects anywhere in the hypothalamic-pituitary-gonadal (HPG) axis can lead to testosterone deficiency. Primary hypogonadism results from primary defects in the testes and is associated with low testosterone levels and elevated levels of gonadotropins. Secondary or hypogonadotropic hypogonadism results from disorders of the hypothalamus and/or pituitary and is associated with low testosterone levels and low or inappropriately low LH and FSH concentrations. The authors review here a stepwise approach to the diagnosis and the epidemiology of androgen deficiency syndromes in men.

PRIMARY HYPOGONADISM

Primary hypogonadism results from congenital or acquired disorders of the testes (**Table 1**). Primary congenital hypogonadism may be due to chromosomal disorders, defects in testosterone biosynthesis, uncorrected cryptorchidism, congenital anorchia, or androgen resistance. Acquired disorders result from external damage to the testes from surgery, trauma, toxins, inflammation, or infection.

Primary Congenital Hypogonadism

Klinefelter syndrome (KS), classically associated with the 47, XXY karyotype, is the most common cause of congenital hypogonadism, affecting one in 660 men[6,7] and is characterized typically by

small, firm testes (<2 mL), low testosterone levels, eunuchoidal proportions, gynecomastia, elevated LH and FSH levels, and impaired spermatogenesis.[8,9] However, there is considerable phenotypic variation due to mosaicism, variable polyglutamine tract length in exon 1 of the androgen receptor or other polymorphisms in the androgen receptor, other genetic factors, and variable testosterone levels; KS may present with learning difficulties and behavioral problems in childhood and with infertility, gynecomastia, or sexual dysfunction in adulthood. Registries of patients with KS have reported higher overall mortality and increased risk of breast cancer, non-Hodgkin lymphomas, lung cancer, and autoimmune diseases, such as systemic lupus erythematosus and Sjögren syndrome, and lower incidence of prostate cancer.[10–12] Although most men with 47, XXY karyotype are azoospermic, pregnancies have been achieved by testicular sperm extraction combined with intracytoplasmic sperm injection.[13–15]

Up to 15% to 20% of patients with KS demonstrate 46, XY/47, XXY mosaicism, which is associated with a milder phenotype. Patients with KS with more than one extra X chromosome have a more severe phenotype, increased risk of congenital malformations, and lower intelligence than individuals with 47, XXY.[16–18] The true prevalence of KS, especially KS mosaicism, may be underestimated as many men with KS remain undiagnosed; a Danish study found that only 25% of adult men with KS had received a diagnosis; of these, less than 10% were diagnosed before puberty.[19]

Structural chromosomal aberrations, including deletions, duplications, and translocations, and other rearrangements can lead to hypogonadism.[20] For example, Noonan syndrome, an autosomal dominant disorder, is caused by a mutation in the *PTPN11* gene and is characterized by dysmorphic facial features, short stature, and heart disease and is associated with abnormal Sertoli and Leydig cell function.[21,22] Leydig cell hypoplasia as a result of LH receptor mutations leads to testosterone deficiency during the first trimester of pregnancy and complete lack of virilization of the external genitalia at birth.[23,24] Additional diagnoses to consider in newborns with 46, XY with ambiguous genitalia include defects of testosterone biosynthesis, 5α-reductase deficiency, or androgen insensitivity due to mutations of the androgen receptor.[25]

Cryptorchidism, if left uncorrected by 2 years of age, predisposes men to an increased risk of infertility, androgen deficiency, and testicular cancer. Cryptorchidism may also be associated with an increased risk of inguinal hernias and testicular torsion.[26] Even unilateral cryptorchidism,

Table 1 Causes of primary hypogonadism	
Primary Congenital	**Primary Acquired**
Klinefelter syndrome	Bilateral testicular trauma/torsion
Other chromosomal abnormalities	Orchiectomy
Noonan syndrome	Cancer chemotherapy and radiation
Defects of testosterone biosynthesis	Bilateral orchitis
Androgen resistance syndromes	Systemic disease
Uncorrected bilateral cryptorchidism	Sickle cell disease
Congenital anorchia	—
Varicocele	—
Myotonic dystrophy	—

corrected before puberty, is associated with decreased sperm count, possibly reflecting unrecognized damage to the fully descended testis or other genetic factors. A growing body of evidence suggests that cryptorchidism, hypospadias, impaired spermatogenesis, and testicular cancer may be related to common genetic and environmental perturbations and are components of the testicular dysgenesis syndrome.[27]

In children with congenital anorchia, the testicular tissue is presumed to have been functioning during fetal life until at least the 16th week of gestation with gonadal regression occurring later; so at birth, sexual differentiation is normal, but the testes are absent and hypogonadism is severe.[28,29] In children presenting as phenotypic boys, in whom testes cannot be palpated in the scrotum, bilateral cryptorchidism can be distinguished from congenital anorchia by the testosterone response to human chorionic gonadotropin (hCG) administration, the measurement of antimüllerian hormone level, and by magnetic resonance of the pelvis and abdomen.

Primary Acquired Hypogonadism

The testes are vulnerable to injury from trauma, torsion, surgery, toxins, infections, inflammation, and systemic diseases. The manifestations of primary acquired hypogonadism depend on the timing of the testicular injury and also on whether spermatogenesis and testosterone secretion are both affected. In general, there is a larger decrease in sperm production than in testosterone secretion because the seminiferous tubules are generally more susceptible to toxins than the Leydig cells. Testicular torsion, which results from twisting of one or both testes on the spermatic cord, leads to acute loss of the blood supply and permanent damage to the seminiferous tubules if not corrected within a few hours. In a nationwide study in the United States, the incidence of testicular torsion among males aged 1 to 25 years was reported to be 4.5 cases per 100,000 persons per year.[30]

Cancer chemotherapeutic agents, especially alkylating agents, such as cyclophosphamide and procarbazine, can cause Leydig cell impairment, damage to the seminiferous tubules, and hypogonadism.[31,32] Testicular germ cells are very sensitive to radiation, and there is a clear relation between radiation dose and testicular damage.[33] Radiation doses of 200 mGy (20 rad) or more are associated with damage to the spermatogonia, and a dose level of 800 mGy (80 rad) is associated with oligospermia or azoospermia; higher doses may completely destroy the germinal epithelium.

Viral orchitis may be caused by the mumps virus, echovirus, lymphocytic choriomeningitis virus, and group B arboviruses. Orchitis occurs in as many as 25% of postpubertal men with mumps; the orchitis is unilateral in about 60% and bilateral in the remainder. Orchitis typically develops a few days after the onset of parotitis. Although testicular function may recover completely in many men after a bout of orchitis, others may experience testicular atrophy. Semen analysis returns to normal in 75% of men with unilateral orchitis but in only about a third of men with bilateral orchitis.[34] Many chronic, systemic diseases, such as cirrhosis, end stage renal disease, and human immunodeficiency virus (HIV) infection, can cause primary hypogonadism.[35-37]

SECONDARY HYPOGONADISM

Secondary hypogonadism can result from congenital or acquired disorders of the hypothalamus or the pituitary (**Table 2**).

Secondary Congenital Hypogonadism

Congenital hypogonadotropic hypogonadism with anosmia (Kallmann syndrome) or without anosmia is a heterogeneous group of disorders that can result from one or more mutations in genes that contribute to the development and migration of the GnRH neurons, olfactory lobe organogenesis, regulation of GnRH secretion, gonadotrope development, or to the regulation of gonadotropin secretion (**Table 3**). Varying patterns of inheritance and penetrance have been described.[38-40] A substantial proportion of patients with idiopathic hypogonadotropic hypogonadism (IHH) may have an oligogenic rather than a monogenic disorder.[41] Patients with complete GnRH deficiency may have complete absence of pubertal development, whereas others may manifest varying degrees of gonadotropin deficiency and pubertal delay; a subset that carries the same mutations as their affected family members may even have normal reproductive function. Complete reversal of gonadotropin deficiency may also occur in adult life after sex steroid therapy in a small proportion of patients with IHH.[38,42] Further, some men with IHH may present with androgen deficiency and infertility in adult life after having gone through apparently normal pubertal development. Nutritional, emotional, or metabolic stressors may unmask gonadotropin deficiency in some patients who harbor mutations in the candidate genes but who previously had normal reproductive function, such as women with hypothalamic amenorrhea. The factors that contribute to the phenotypic variation in IHH are incompletely

Table 2
Causes of secondary hypogonadism

Secondary Congenital	Secondary Acquired
Idiopathic hypogonadotropic hypogonadism with or without anosmia	Hyperprolactinemia
Gonadotropin or gonadotropin receptor mutations	Medications (GnRH analogues, steroids, opioids)
Leptin or leptin receptor mutations	Critical illness
DAX1 mutations	Severe obesity
PC1 mutations	Eating disorders
Prader Willi syndrome	*Damage to gonadotroph cells* Tumors Infiltrative diseases (sarcoidosis, Langerhans cell histiocytosis, hemochromatosis) Infection Pituitary apoplexy Trauma

understood, but oligogenicity and gene-gene and gene-environment interactions are likely contributors.[38,41,42]

The incidence of congenital hypogonadotropic hypogonadism is approximately 1 to 10:100,000 live births (IHH).[43,44] Mutations in a large number of genes, including GnRH1/GnRHR, TAC3/TACR3, FGF8/FGF17, PROK2/PROKR2, NELF, CHD7, HS6ST1, WDR11, SEMA3A, SOX10, IL17RD2, DUSP6, SPRY4, and FLRT3, have been implicated in the genesis of IHH; this list continues to grow.[45] Mutations of the Dax1 gene lead to hypogonadism associated with congenital adrenal hypoplasia.[46] Mutations in the prohormone convertase gene lead to hypogonadism in conjunction with severe obesity, hypocortisolism, and diabetes.[47] Similarly, leptin or leptin receptor mutations lead to morbid obesity along with hypogonadotropic hypogonadism.[48] The defect may rarely lie above the level of the hypothalamus; kisspeptin stimulates GnRH neurons in the hypothalamus to secrete GnRH, and mutations in the kisspeptin receptor lead to congenital hypogonadotropic hypogonadism.[49,50] Mutations of the gonadotropins and their receptors have also been described with varying consequences on

Table 3
Genes associated with idiopathic hypogonadotropic hypogonadism

Inheritance	Gene	Loss of Function Phenotype
X-linked	Kal1	HH + anosmia
	DAX1	HH + adrenal insufficiency
Autosomal dominant	FGFR1	Autosomal dominant form of HH
Autosomal recessive	GnRHR	HH, poor response to GnRH
	KISS1R	Impaired GnRH secretion
	SF1	Sex reversal + adrenal insufficiency
	NELF	HH + anosmia
	Prok2, Prok2R	HH + anosmia
	Tac3, Tac3R	HH
	Leptin	Obesity + HH
	Leptin R	Obesity + HH
	GnRH	Hpg mouse, IHH, one case of human mutation
	CHD7	Anosmia, other features of CHARGE syndrome

Abbreviations: CHD7, CHARGE syndrome locus: eye coloboma, choanal atresia, growth and developmental retardation, genitourinary anomalies, ear anomalies; DAX1, dosage-sensitive sex-reversal, adrenal hypoplasia congenita, X-chromosome; FGFR1, fibroblast growth factor receptor 1; GnRHR, GnRH receptor; HH, Hypogonadotropic hypogonadism; HPG, hypogonadal; KAL1, interval-1 gene; KISS1R, kisspeptin 1 receptor; LEP, leptin; leptin R, leptin receptor; NELF, nasal embryonic LHRH factor; PROK2, prokineticin 2; Prok2R, prokineticin 2 receptor; SF1, steroidogenic factor 1; Tac3, tachykinin 3; Tac3R, tachykinin 3 receptor.

reproductive health.[51] Mutations in homeodomain transcription factors, such as *Prop1*, *Pit1*, *Hsx1*, and others may be associated with failure of differentiation of one or more pituitary cell lineage resulting in deficiency of one or more pituitary hormones.[52]

Secondary Acquired Hypogonadism

Hypogonadotropic hypogonadism can be caused by any disease process that affects the HPG axis by suppressing GnRH secretion from the hypothalamus, preventing GnRH from reaching the pituitary by stalk injury, and damaging the pituitary itself, effectively lowering the secretion of the gonadotropins. Hyperprolactinemia can suppress GnRH secretion and gonadotropin response to GnRH secretion, resulting in suppressed LH and FSH secretion and consequently in low testosterone levels.[53,54]

The HPG axis is sensitive to alterations in energy balance, emotional or physiologic stress, and illness.[55] Hypogonadotropic hypogonadism may be the primary intent of a medication (ie, GnRH analogues used in the treatment of prostate cancer) or an undesired consequence of medications, including androgenic anabolic steroids, glucocorticoids, marijuana, and chronic opiates. SHBG levels are negatively associated with body mass index; therefore, men with mild to moderate obesity typically have low total testosterone levels but normal free testosterone levels. Severe obesity may be associated with true hypogonadotropic hypogonadism in which both total and free testosterone levels are suppressed.[56] Eating disorders are less common in men than in women and can be associated with hypogonadism.[57] Damage to the gonadotroph cells can result from both benign and malignant tumors, infiltrative diseases (ie, sarcoidosis, Langerhans cell histiocytosis, hemochromatosis), infection, and pituitary apoplexy, which may be spontaneous or due to trauma; the hypogonadism may be transient or permanent.

Chronic opioid use is emerging as an important cause of secondary hypogonadism and has been associated with an increased risk of sexual dysfunction, osteoporosis, and fractures in men.[58–61] Typically, 20 mg of methadone or equivalent doses of other opiates are sufficient to suppress testosterone levels.[58–61]

After prolonged use of large doses of anabolic-androgenic steroid (AAS), the recovery of HPT axis may take a long time, be incomplete, or may not occur at all leading to AAS withdrawal hypogonadism.[62–64] In some men's health clinics, AAS withdrawal hypogonadism has emerged as an important cause of androgen deficiency.[63,64] In a retrospective review of 6033 patients attending a men's health clinic in Texas,[64] 43% of those with total testosterone less than 50 ng/dL reported prior AAS exposure. In another report, 21% of 382 hypogonadal men seeking testosterone replacement therapy had earlier AAS exposure.

EPIDEMIOLOGY OF HYPOGONADISM

The prevalence and incidence of organic hypogonadism in men due to known diseases of the testes, pituitary, and the hypothalamus remain unknown. Only a small fraction of men receiving testosterone therapy in the United States have a known condition of the testes, pituitary, and the hypothalamus.[65,66] Surveys of testosterone use in the United States have found that men between 50 and 70 years of age are the most frequent recipients of testosterone prescription.[65,66] This finding suggests that a sizable proportion of testosterone therapy is being prescribed for age-related decline in testosterone levels, for which testosterone therapy is not approved. Prescription opioid use and AAS use are emerging as important contributors to men receiving a testosterone prescription in the United States. The presence of comorbid conditions, such as obesity, obstructive sleep apnea, depression, and diabetes, and use of antidepressants or systemic glucocorticoids are associated with an increased likelihood of testosterone prescription.

Many epidemiologic studies have estimated the prevalence of age-related decline in testosterone levels. These prevalence estimates have varied because of heterogeneity of the study populations, the definition of low testosterone, and the assay used to measure circulating testosterone concentrations.[67–70] These studies are in agreement that testosterone levels decline gradually with advancing age without a clear inflection point or andropause. As SHBG levels increase with age, the free testosterone levels decline with a steeper trajectory than total testosterone levels. The age-related decline in testosterone levels is due to defects at all levels of the hypothalamic-pituitary-testicular axis; the trajectory of decline is affected by body mass index, weight gain, comorbid conditions, medications, and genetic factors.[71]

The term *late-onset hypogonadism* reflects the viewpoint that in some middle-aged and older men, the age-related decline in testosterone is associated with a cluster of symptoms and signs that resemble those observed in men with classic androgen deficiency.[68] In an analysis of the European Male Aging Study, sexual symptoms (poor morning erection, low sexual desire, and erectile dysfunction) were associated with testosterone levels less than 320 ng/dL (11 nmol/L) or free testosterone less than 64 pg/mL (220 pmol/L).[68] The men defined as having late-onset hypogonadism by these criteria tended to be older and had higher body mass index; lower muscle mass, bone mineral density, and hemoglobin; and slower gait speed than those who had normal testosterone levels. Recent studies, using the liquid chromatography tandem mass spectrometry (LC-MS/MS) assay for the measurement of total testosterone concentrations in early morning samples, have reported a 10% to 14% prevalence of low testosterone levels in community-dwelling men 65 years of age or older.[67–70] In the European Male Aging Study, the prevalence of late-onset hypogonadism defined by symptoms and total testosterone less than 220 ng/dL (8 nmol/L) was 3.2% for men aged 60 to 69 years and 5.1% for those aged 70 to 79 years.[67]

Testosterone and Metabolic Disorders

In epidemiologic studies, low total testosterone levels have been associated with an increased risk of diabetes and metabolic syndrome. However, in longitudinal analyses of epidemiologic data, SHBG levels, but not total or free testosterone levels, are independently associated with incident diabetes and metabolic syndrome after adjusting for age, adiposity, and comorbid conditions.[72,73] SHBG is being recognized as an important independent marker of metabolic risk.

The induction of severe acute deficiency of testosterone, such as that induced by withdrawal of testosterone therapy in men with IHH or that induced therapeutically in men with prostate cancer receiving androgen deprivation therapy, is associated with the worsening of insulin resistance.[74,75] Furthermore, testosterone administration reduces whole-body, subcutaneous as well as visceral fat[76]; therefore, testosterone therapy would be expected to improve insulin resistance in androgen-deficient men. However, randomized clinical trials have not shown consistent improvements in insulin resistance or diabetes outcomes with testosterone therapy.

Although several randomized, placebo-controlled trials of testosterone have been conducted in men with diabetes, the results of only one such trial have been published. The TIMES2 (Testosterone Replacement in Hypogonadal Men With Type 2 Diabetes and/or Metabolic Syndrome) Study was a randomized trial in which men with type 2 diabetes and/or metabolic syndrome were randomized to either 2% testosterone gel or placebo gel for 6 months.[77] The change in hemoglobin A1C between groups did not differ significantly between groups. Thus, this and other unpublished trials have failed to show significant improvements in diabetes outcomes with testosterone therapy, although some trials have reported improvements in homeostatic model assessment for insulin resistance (HOMA-IR).

DIAGNOSIS OF ANDROGEN DEFICIENCY SYNDROMES IN MEN
Who Should Be Screened for Androgen Deficiency?

General population screening for male hypogonadism is not recommended.[1] Instead, the Endocrine Society recommends screening in men who have conditions in which there is a high prevalence of low testosterone levels[1]: those presenting with sexual dysfunction, infertility, gynecomastia, sellar mass, radiation to the sellar region, or other diseases of the sellar region; those who have received treatment with medications that affect testosterone production or metabolism, such as AASs, glucocorticoids, and opioids; men with HIV with weight loss; and those with osteoporosis or low-trauma fracture, especially at a young age (**Box 1**).

Patient History

The Endocrine Society recommends making a diagnosis of androgen deficiency only in men with consistent signs and symptoms and unequivocally low serum testosterone levels.[1] Therefore, an important first step in the diagnostic workup

---

Box 1
Who should be screened for androgen deficiency?

The Endocrine Society recommends screening men at increased risk of having low testosterone levels, such as those presenting with

- Sexual dysfunction
- Infertility
- Gynecomastia
- Sellar mass, radiation to the sellar region, or other diseases of the sellar region
- Treatment with medications that affect testosterone production or metabolism, such as anabolic-androgenic steroids, glucocorticoids, and opioids
- Men with HIV with weight loss
- Osteoporosis or low-trauma fracture, especially at a young age

of androgen deficiency in men is the ascertainment of symptoms and a general health evaluation to exclude systemic disorders; eating disorders; excessive exercise; use of drugs that suppress testosterone production or action, such as opioids, GnRH agonists or antagonists, antiandrogens, glucocorticoids, or spironolactone; use of drugs of abuse, such as marijuana, AASs, excessive use of alcohol, and opioids. History should ascertain the patients' developmental milestones of sexual development, current symptoms, lifestyle factors, medications, and information about possible causes of hypogonadism. Adolescents and young adults who have not yet completed puberty may report small genitalia, difficulty gaining muscle mass, lack of a need to shave, and failure of the voice to deepen. Adult men may present with decreased libido, difficulty with erections, low energy, low mood, gynecomastia, or infertility. In middle-aged and older men, there is considerable overlap between age-related symptoms and those due to androgen deficiency. In the European Male Aging study (EMAS), 3 sexual symptoms, including poor morning erections, low libido, and erectile dysfunction, were shown to have a syndromic association with decreased testosterone levels.[68] Gynecomastia is more likely to occur in primary than in secondary hypogonadism.

Many validated questionnaires have been developed to aid in the diagnosis of hypogonadism; but the specificity of these questionnaires is low, and their use is not recommended.[78,79]

Physical Examination

The physical signs of hypogonadism depend on the age of onset of androgen deficiency (**Table 4**),

the severity of testosterone deficiency, and whether or not there is impaired spermatogenesis. Androgen deficiency in the first trimester of fetal life results in varying degrees of genital ambiguity. Testosterone deficiency occurring later in gestation can cause cryptorchidism and micropenis. Prepubertal hypogonadism is associated with failure to develop secondary sexual characteristics resulting in failure of penile and scrotal enlargement and pigmentation; deepening of the voice; appropriate pubic, facial, and body hair development; and temporal recession of the hairline. Men with prepubertal onset of androgen deficiency may have female pattern escutcheon and eunuchoidal skeletal proportions (a lower body segment that is more than 2 cm longer than upper body segment and an arm span that is more than 5 cm longer than height) because of delayed closure of the epiphyseal plates in long bones. In comparison, a normal adult man has approximately equal upper and lower body segments as well as nearly equal arm span and height.

Physical examination should ascertain hair growth, body proportions, penile length, location of urethral meatus, testicular volume, the presence of breast enlargement, and any dysmorphic features. Testicular size should be measured using a Prader orchidometer. Adult men normally have a testicular volume greater than 15 mL. The flaccid penis should be examined for the presence of hypospadias, epispadias, and chordee. The average flaccid penile length is 9.2 cm; a micropenis is defined as the penile length 2.5 SDs less than the mean, which is less than 5.2 cm in flaccid and less than 8.5 cm in the

Table 4
Signs of fetal, prepubertal, and postpubertal onset of hypogonadism

Fetal Development	Prepuberty	Postpubertal
Eunuchoidal stature	Eunuchoidal stature	Normal stature
Female or ambiguous genitalia	Small testes (usually <6 cm³)	Testes volume normal to slightly low (>10 cm³); soft
Small testes (usually <6 cm³)	Small penis (<5 cm) Lack of normal scrotal rugae and pigmentation	Penis normal size Normal scrotal rugae and pigmentation
Small penis (<5 cm)	Small prostate	Normal prostate
Lack of normal scrotal rugae and pigmentation	Scant facial, axillary, and pubic hair	Thinning of facial, axillary, and pubic hair
Small prostate	High voice	Normal voice
Scant facial, axillary, and pubic hair	Lack of male pattern baldness	Lack of male pattern baldness
High voice	—	—

stretched penis.[80] The epididymis and vas deferens should be examined to assess for the presence of a varicocele, which can be palpated along the posterior portion of the cord.

Androgen deficiency before puberty may be associated with diminished facial and body hair and a female pattern escutcheon, but axillary and pubic hair may develop because of the effects of adrenal androgens. The development of androgen deficiency after puberty is associated with diminished facial or body hair. Severe hypogonadism of longstanding duration may be associated with the classic hypogonadal facies (pallor and fine wrinkling around the mouth and eyes), altered femininelike fat distribution, and gynecomastia.

LABORATORY TESTING

The next step is the measurement of serum total testosterone concentration in an early morning fasting sample (**Fig. 1**A) using a reliable assay preferably in a Centers for Disease Control and Prevention (CDC)–certified laboratory. Testosterone concentrations vary greatly among men and within the same person over time. For instance, in the Boston Area Community Health Study, 21% of men whose initial testosterone concentration was

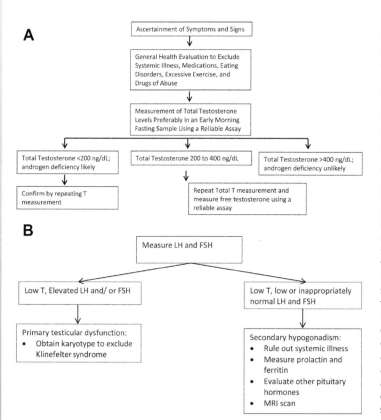

Fig. 1. (A) A stepwise approach to the diagnostic workup of men suspected of having androgen deficiency. The diagnostic workup of men suspected of having androgen deficiency can be conceptualized as a multistep process that starts with ascertainment of symptoms and signs of androgen deficiency and general health evaluation to exclude systemic illness, medications that can affect testosterone production or action, drugs of abuse that can affect testosterone production or action, eating disorders, and excessive exercise. The next step is the measurement of serum total testosterone concentrations in a fasting early morning blood sample using a reliable assay, such as a Centers for Disease Control and Prevention–certified LC-MS/MS assay. If total testosterone concentration is very low (<200 ng/dL) in an assay with the lower limit at approximately 300 ng/dL, then androgen deficiency is very likely and the diagnosis should be confirmed by repeating the measurement. If testosterone concentration is greater than 400 ng/dL in an assay with a lower limit of the normal range at approximately 300 ng/dL, then androgen deficiency is unlikely. In men with total testosterone concentration in the borderline range of 200 to 400 ng/dL, total testosterone should be repeated and free testosterone level should also be measured using a reliable assay. The men deemed to be androgen deficient should then have LH and FSH measured to determine whether the defect resides at the testicular level or at the level of the hypothalamus and the pituitary as shown in B. (B) Further workup of men deemed to be androgen deficient. In men deemed to be androgen deficient, measurement of LH and FSH concentrations can help distinguish primary from secondary hypogonadism. Obtain karyotype in men with primary testicular dysfunction to exclude KS, which is the most common cause of primary testicular dysfunction. In patients with secondary hypogonadism, measure prolactin and ferritin to exclude hyperprolactinemia, evaluate other pituitary hormones, and an MRI scan to rule out space-occupying lesions of the pituitary and the hypothalamic region. By excluding other organic causes of hypogonadotropic hypogonadism, one is left with a diagnosis of IHH. IHH is a heterogeneous group of disorders; the presence of associated dysmorphic features, such as anosmia, synkinesia, or hyperphagia, can help identify the specific syndrome. T, testosterone.

less than 300 ng/dL had normal testosterone concentration on subsequent testing on a different day.[81] Thus, the diagnosis of androgen deficiency should not be made based on a single low testosterone level.

Some of the variation in testosterone levels in men is due to biological factors, such as pulsatile, diurnal, and circannual rhythms of testosterone secretion; genetic factors; and variations in sex hormone binding globulin concentrations; some of the variation is due to methodological problems, such as interassay and interlaboratory variations and calibrator differences.[82] Heritable factors contribute to the population level variation in testosterone levels. Polymorphisms in the SHBG gene and in an X chromosome locus have been associated with variation in testosterone levels in men.[83]

Total testosterone represents the sum of unbound testosterone and that which is bound testosterone to plasma proteins (**Fig. 2**A) and can be measured by immunoassays, immunometric assays, and by LC-MS/MS. Many platform-based immunoassays and immunometric assays lack accuracy, especially in the low range prevalent in hypogonadal men. The LC-MS/MS assays

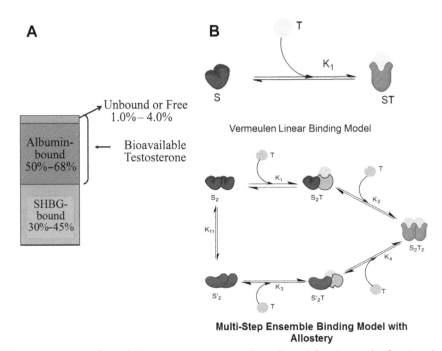

Fig. 2. (*A*) The partitioning of circulating testosterone into the unbound fraction and a fraction that is bound mostly to albumin and SHBG, and the concept of free and bioavailable testosterone. Circulating testosterone is bound to SHBG (30%–45%) and to human serum albumin (50%–68%). 1% to 4% of circulating testosterone is unbound or free and can be measured using equilibrium dialysis. Some evidence suggests that albumin-bound testosterone, being loosely bound with low affinity, can dissociate at the capillary level, especially in tissues with long transit time, such as the liver and brain. This finding has led to the concept that albumin-bound plus unbound testosterone is bioavailable; this bioavailable testosterone fraction can be measured using the ammonium sulfate precipitation method. (*B*) The Vermeulen linear model of testosterone binding to SHBG and the new multistep binding model with allostery. The old linear model of testosterone's binding to SHBG assumes that one molecule of testosterone binds one molecule of SHBG with a single binding affinity. However, recent experimental evidence indicates that SHBG circulates as a dimer and that the binding of testosterone to SHBG is a complex, multistep process, characterized by ground state heterogeneity in SHBG isoforms. The binding of the first testosterone molecule to the first binding site on SHBG dimer leads to a conformational rearrangement and allosteric interaction between the binding sites such that the second testosterone molecule binds to the second binding site with a different binding affinity. The multistep binding model with allostery provides estimates of free testosterone that closely approximate those measured using equilibrium dialysis. K, dissociation constant; S, SHBG; ST, SHBG-bound testosterone; T, testosterone. ([*B*] *Adapted from* Vermeulen A, Verdonck L, Kaufman JM. A critical evaluation of simple methods for the estimation of free testosterone in serum. J Clin Endocrinol Metab 1999;84(10):3666–72; and Zakharov MN, Bhasin S, Travison TG, et al. A multi-step, dynamic allosteric model of testosterone's binding to sex hormone binding globulin. Mol Cell Endocrinol 2015;399:193, with permission.)

involve extraction of steroids from the serum using organic reagents, chromatographic separation of testosterone from other steroids by high-performance liquid chromatography and mass spectrometry, followed by detection of specific fragments of testosterone by mass spectrometry. Liquid chromatography tandem mass spectrometry (LC-MS/MS) has emerged as the reference method with the highest accuracy and precision. Many LC-MS/MS–based assays for testosterone are now available from several commercial laboratories. With the availability of testosterone calibrators from the National Institutes of Standards and Technologies and the CDC's Hormone Standardization Program for Testosterone, the interlaboratory variation in LC-MS/MS–based assays in CDC-certified laboratories has decreased substantially.

Total testosterone concentrations are affected by the circulating concentrations of SHBG; therefore, measurement of free testosterone levels is important in conditions in which alterations in circulating SHBG concentrations may be expected, such as obesity, diabetes mellitus, old age, HIV infection, acromegaly, liver and kidney diseases, and hypothyroidism and hyperthyroidism (**Box 2**). Free testosterone concentrations can be measured using equilibrium dialysis and ultrafiltration, or estimated from total testosterone, SHBG, and albumin concentrations. Free testosterone measurements by tracer analogue methods have consistently been found to be inaccurate and are not recommended.[5] The linear law-of-mass actions for estimating free testosterone concentrations are based on assumptions of linear testosterone binding of testosterone to SHBG with a single binding constant (see **Fig. 2B**)[84]; these assumptions have recently been shown to be inaccurate.[1,84] Recent studies have shown that SHBG exists as a dimer in human circulation and that the binding of testosterone to SHBG is a complex, multi-step process involving ground state heterogeneity in circulating SHBG molecules and allosteric interaction between the two binding sites on the SHBG dimer such that the binding affinities of the two binding sites are not equivalent (see **Fig. 2B**).[85] The estimates of free testosterone concentration using this new multistep ensemble binding model with allostery provide close approximation to those measured using equilibrium dialysis.[85]

Reference ranges for testosterone vary among laboratories so physicians should use the lower limit specific to the assay and the laboratory.[86] Reference ranges provided by most laboratories are typically based on small convenience samples or hospital-based patients. In a recent study, the 2.5th percentile value for healthy, nonobese young men, 19 to 40 years of age, in the Framingham Heart Study was 348 ng/dL. The efforts to generate population-based reference ranges harmonized across various geographic regions are currently in progress. There is no consensus on the exact level of testosterone that defines hypogonadism; but in healthy young men, in many research laboratories, the lower limit of normal for total testosterone tends to be 280 to 300 ng/dL (9.8–10.4 nmol/L) and for free testosterone 70 to 90 pg/mL (0.24–0.31 nmol/L) by equilibrium dialysis.[1]

In men deemed to be androgen deficient, measurement of LH and FSH concentrations can help to distinguish between primary and secondary hypogonadism. In secondary hypogonadism, a normal or low-normal LH is inappropriate in the setting of a low testosterone level (see **Fig. 1**). If secondary hypogonadism is detected, a prolactin level should be obtained to rule out hyperprolactinemia, serum iron and total iron binding capacity measured to rule out hemochromatosis, and dedicated pituitary imaging with an MRI to rule out a space-occupying lesion (see **Fig. 1B**). hCG stimulation and GnRH stimulation tests are rarely used today to establish the diagnosis of androgen deficiency.

Box 2
Conditions with alterations in circulating SHBG concentrations

Conditions in which SHBG concentrations are increased

- Old age
- Chronic infections, such as HIV and hepatitis C virus
- Hyperthyroidism
- Acromegaly
- Estrogen therapy
- Use of anticonvulsants
- Hepatitis

Conditions in which SHBG concentrations are decreased

- Obesity
- Diabetes mellitus
- Metabolic syndrome
- Hypothyroidism
- Medications: androgen therapy, glucocorticoids, progestins
- Advanced liver disease
- Nephrotic syndrome

Semen Analysis

The semen analysis is necessary for the assessment of male fertility. The standard semen analysis consists of measuring the following parameters: semen volume, pH, sperm concentration, motility, morphology, leukocyte count, search for immature germ cells, and microscopy for debris and agglutination. Semen should be collected by masturbation after 48 to 72 hours of sexual abstinence, and the specimen should be examined within 1 hour after collection. The World Health Organization has generated the following one-sided reference limits for semen parameters[87]: semen volume, 1.5 mL; total sperm number, 39 million per ejaculate; sperm concentration, 15 million per milliliter; vitality, 58% live; progressive motility, 32%; total (progressive + nonprogressive) motility, 40%; morphologically normal forms, 4.0%. A variety of tests for sperm function can be performed in specialized laboratories, but these add little to the treatment options.

SUMMARY/DISCUSSION

The diagnosis of hypogonadism is made by ascertainment of signs and symptoms and demonstration of consistently low testosterone levels on 2 or more occasions using a reliable assay. The nonspecificity of symptoms, substantial variations in testosterone levels due to biological factors, poor precision and accuracy of many immunoassays, and poorly defined reference ranges contribute to increased risk of misclassification. The use of reliable assays, preferably LC-MS/MS assays in a CDC-certified laboratory, for testosterone measurement; rigorously derived reference ranges; and the use of ancillary data, such as testicular volume and LH and FSH concentrations, can greatly reduce the risk of misclassification.

REFERENCES

1. Bhasin S, Cunningham GR, Hayes FJ, et al. Testosterone therapy in men with androgen deficiency syndromes: an Endocrine Society clinical practice guideline. J Clin Endocrinol Metab 2010;95(6): 2536–59.
2. Hammond GL, Bocchinfuso WP. Sex hormone-binding globulin: gene organization and structure/function analyses. Horm Res 1996;45(3–5): 197–201.
3. Mendel CM. The free hormone hypothesis: a physiologically based mathematical model. Endocr Rev 1989;10(3):232–74.
4. Rosner W. Plasma steroid-binding proteins. Endocrinol Metab Clin North Am 1991;20(4):697–720.
5. Rosner W, Auchus RJ, Azziz R, et al. Position statement: utility, limitations, and pitfalls in measuring testosterone: an Endocrine Society position statement. J Clin Endocrinol Metab 2007;92(2):405–13.
6. Bojesen A, Gravholt CH. Klinefelter syndrome in clinical practice. Nat Clin Pract Urol 2007;4(4):192–204.
7. Groth KA, Skakkebæk A, Høst C, et al. Clinical review: Klinefelter syndrome–a clinical update. J Clin Endocrinol Metab 2013;98(1):20–30.
8. Lanfranco F, Kamischke A, Zitzmann M, et al. Klinefelter's syndrome. Lancet 2004;364(9430): 273–83.
9. Paduch DA, Fine RG, Bolyakov A, et al. New concepts in Klinefelter syndrome. Curr Opin Urol 2008; 18(6):621–7.
10. Swerdlow AJ, Schoemaker MJ, Higgins CD, et al, UK Clinical Cytogenetics Group. Cancer incidence and mortality in men with Klinefelter syndrome: a cohort study. J Natl Cancer Inst 2005;97(16): 1204–10.
11. Swerdlow AJ, Higgins CD, Schoemaker MJ, et al, United Kingdom Clinical Cytogenetics Group. Mortality in patients with Klinefelter syndrome in Britain: a cohort study. J Clin Endocrinol Metab 2005; 90(12):6516–22.
12. Bojesen A, Gravholt CH. Morbidity and mortality in Klinefelter syndrome (47,XXY). Acta Paediatr 2011; 100(6):807–13.
13. Plotton I, Giscard d'Estaing S, Cuzin B, et al, FERTIPRESERVE group. Preliminary results of a prospective study of testicular sperm extraction in young versus adult patients with nonmosaic 47,XXY Klinefelter syndrome. J Clin Endocrinol Metab 2015;100(3):961–7.
14. Greco E, Scarselli F, Minasi MG, et al. Birth of 16 healthy children after ICSI in cases of nonmosaic Klinefelter syndrome. Hum Reprod 2013;28(5): 1155–60.
15. Madureira C, Cunha M, Sousa M, et al. Treatment by testicular sperm extraction and intracytoplasmic sperm injection of 65 azoospermic patients with non-mosaic Klinefelter syndrome with birth of 17 healthy children. Andrology 2014;2(4):623–31.
16. Abdelmoula NB, Amouri A, Portnoi MF, et al. Cytogenetics and fluorescence in situ hybridization assessment of sex-chromosome mosaicism in Klinefelter's syndrome. Ann Genet 2004;47(2):163–75.
17. Fruhmesser A, Kotzot D. Chromosomal variants in Klinefelter syndrome. Sex Dev 2011;5(3):109–23.
18. Tartaglia N, Ayari N, Howell S, et al. 48,XXYY, 48,XXXY and 49,XXXXY syndromes: not just variants of Klinefelter syndrome. Acta Paediatr 2011;100(6): 851–60.
19. Bojesen A, Juul S, Gravholt CH. Prenatal and postnatal prevalence of Klinefelter syndrome: a national registry study. J Clin Endocrinol Metab 2003;88(2): 622–6.

20. Maduro MR, Lamb DJ. Understanding new genetics of male infertility. J Urol 2002;168(5): 2197–205.

21. Ankarberg-Lindgren C, Westphal O, Dahlgren J. Testicular size development and reproductive hormones in boys and adult males with Noonan syndrome: a longitudinal study. Eur J Endocrinol 2011; 165(1):137–44.

22. Tartaglia M, Mehler EL, Goldberg R, et al. Mutations in PTPN11, encoding the protein tyrosine phosphatase SHP-2, cause Noonan syndrome. Nat Genet 2001;29(4):465–8.

23. Latronico AC, Anasti J, Arnhold IJ, et al. Brief report: testicular and ovarian resistance to luteinizing hormone caused by inactivating mutations of the luteinizing hormone-receptor gene. N Engl J Med 1996;334(8):507–12.

24. Aaronson IA. Micropenis: medical and surgical implications. J Urol 1994;152(1):4–14.

25. Krishnan S, Wisniewski AB. Ambiguous genitalia in the newborn. 2000.

26. Docimo SG, Silver RI, Cromie W. The undescended testicle: diagnosis and management. Am Fam Physician 2000;62(9):2037–44, 2047–8.

27. Sharpe RM, Skakkebaek NE. Testicular dysgenesis syndrome: mechanistic insights and potential new downstream effects. Fertil Steril 2008;89(2 Suppl): e33–8.

28. Abeyaratne MR, Aherne WA, Scott JE. The vanishing testis. Lancet 1969;2(7625):822–4.

29. Aynsley-Green A, Zachmann M, Illig R, et al. Congenital bilateral anorchia in childhood: a clinical, endocrine and therapeutic evaluation of twenty-one cases. Clin Endocrinol (Oxf) 1976;5(4):381–91.

30. Mansbach JM, Forbes P, Peters C. Testicular torsion and risk factors for orchiectomy. Arch Pediatr Adolesc Med 2005;159(12):1167–71.

31. Nord C, Bjøro T, Ellingsen D, et al. Gonadal hormones in long-term survivors 10 years after treatment for unilateral testicular cancer. Eur Urol 2003; 44(3):322–8.

32. Friedman NM, Plymate SR. Leydig cell dysfunction and gynaecomastia in adult males treated with alkylating agents. Clin Endocrinol (Oxf) 1980;12(6):553–6.

33. Rowley MJ, Leach DR, Warner GA, et al. Effect of graded doses of ionizing radiation on the human testis. Radiat Res 1974;59(3):665–78.

34. Aiman J, Brenner PF, MacDonald PC. Androgen and estrogen production in elderly men with gynecomastia and testicular atrophy after mumps orchitis. J Clin Endocrinol Metab 1980;50(2):380–6.

35. Holdsworth S, Atkins RC, de Kretser DM. The pituitary-testicular axis in men with chronic renal failure. N Engl J Med 1977;296(22):1245–9.

36. Baker HW, Burger HG, de Kretser DM, et al. A study of the endocrine manifestations of hepatic cirrhosis. Q J Med 1976;45(177):145–78.

37. Rochira V, Diazzi C, Santi D, et al. Low testosterone is associated with poor health status in men with human immunodeficiency virus infection: a retrospective study. Andrology 2015;3(2):298–308.

38. Pitteloud N, Quinton R, Pearce S, et al. Digenic mutations account for variable phenotypes in idiopathic hypogonadotropic hypogonadism. J Clin Invest 2007;117(2):457–63.

39. Sykiotis GP, Plummer L, Hughes VA, et al. Oligogenic basis of isolated gonadotropin-releasing hormone deficiency. Proc Natl Acad Sci U S A 2010;107(34):15140–4.

40. Seminara SB, Oliveira LM, Beranova M, et al. Genetics of hypogonadotropic hypogonadism. J Endocrinol Invest 2000;23(9):560–5.

41. Balasubramanian R, Dwyer A, Seminara SB, et al. Human GnRH deficiency: a unique disease model to unravel the ontogeny of GnRH neurons. Neuroendocrinology 2010;92(2):81–99.

42. Mitchell AL, Dwyer A, Pitteloud N, et al. Genetic basis and variable phenotypic expression of Kallmann syndrome: towards a unifying theory. Trends Endocrinol Metab 2011;22(7):249–58.

43. Fraietta R, Zylberstejn DS, Esteves SC. Hypogonadotropic hypogonadism revisited. Clinics (Sao Paulo) 2013;68(Suppl 1):81–8.

44. Salenave S, Chanson P, Bry H, et al. Kallmann's syndrome: a comparison of the reproductive phenotypes in men carrying KAL1 and FGFR1/KAL2 mutations. J Clin Endocrinol Metab 2008; 93(3):758–63.

45. Ghervan C, Young J. Congenital hypogonadotropic hypogonadism and Kallmann syndrome in males. Presse Med 2014;43(2):152–61 [in French].

46. Burris TP, Guo W, McCabe ER. The gene responsible for adrenal hypoplasia congenita, DAX-1, encodes a nuclear hormone receptor that defines a new class within the superfamily. Recent Prog Horm Res 1996;51:241–59 [discussion: 259–60].

47. Jackson RS, Creemers JW, Ohagi S, et al. Obesity and impaired prohormone processing associated with mutations in the human prohormone convertase 1 gene. Nat Genet 1997;16(3):303–6.

48. Strobel A, Issad T, Camoin L, et al. A leptin missense mutation associated with hypogonadism and morbid obesity. Nat Genet 1998;18(3):213–5.

49. Messager S, Chatzidaki EE, Ma D, et al. Kisspeptin directly stimulates gonadotropin-releasing hormone release via G protein-coupled receptor 54. Proc Natl Acad Sci U S A 2005;102(5):1761–6.

50. Seminara SB, Messager S, Chatzidaki EE, et al. The GPR54 gene as a regulator of puberty. N Engl J Med 2003;349(17):1614–27.

51. Themmen APN, Huhtaniemi IT. Mutations of gonadotropins and gonadotropin receptors: elucidating the physiology and pathophysiology of pituitary-gonadal function. Endocr Rev 2000;21(5):551–83.

52. Parks JS, Brown MR, Hurley DL, et al. Heritable disorders of pituitary development. J Clin Endocrinol Metab 1999;84(12):4362–70.

53. Carter JN, Tyson JE, Tolis G, et al. Prolactin-screening tumors and hypogonadism in 22 men. N Engl J Med 1978;299(16):847–52.

54. Maggi M, Buvat J, Corona G, et al. Hormonal causes of male sexual dysfunctions and their management (hyperprolactinemia, thyroid disorders, GH disorders, and DHEA). J Sex Med 2013;10(3):661–77.

55. Rolih CA, Ober KP. The endocrine response to critical illness. Med Clin North Am 1995;79(1):211–24.

56. Dandona P, Dhindsa S. Update: hypogonadotropic hypogonadism in type 2 diabetes and obesity. J Clin Endocrinol Metab 2011;96(9):2643–51.

57. Winston AP, Wijeratne S. Hypogonadism, hypoleptinaemia and osteoporosis in males with eating disorders. Clin Endocrinol (Oxf) 2009;71(6):897–8.

58. Hallinan R, Byrne A, Agho K, et al. Hypogonadism in men receiving methadone and buprenorphine maintenance treatment. Int J Androl 2009;32(2):131–9.

59. Yee A, Loh HS, Hisham Hashim HM, et al. The prevalence of sexual dysfunction among male patients on methadone and buprenorphine treatments: a meta-analysis study. J Sex Med 2014; 11(1):22–32.

60. Li L, Setoguchi S, Cabral H, et al. Opioid use for noncancer pain and risk of fracture in adults: a nested case-control study using the general practice research database. Am J Epidemiol 2013; 178(4):559–69.

61. Kim TW, Alford DP, Malabanan A, et al. Low bone density in patients receiving methadone maintenance treatment. Drug Alcohol Depend 2006;85(3): 258–62.

62. Kanayama G, Hudson JI, DeLuca J, et al. Prolonged hypogonadism in males following withdrawal from anabolic-androgenic steroids: an under-recognized problem. Addiction 2015;110(5):823–31.

63. Coward RM, Rajanahally S, Kovac JR, et al. Anabolic steroid induced hypogonadism in young men. J Urol 2013;190(6):2200–5.

64. Rahnema CD, Lipshultz LI, Crosnoe LE, et al. Anabolic steroid-induced hypogonadism: diagnosis and treatment. Fertil Steril 2014;101(5):1271–9.

65. Jasuja GK, Bhasin S, Reisman JI, et al. Ascertainment of testosterone prescribing practices in the VA. Med Care 2015 Sep;53(9):746–52.

66. Nguyen CP, Hirsch MS, Moeny D, et al. Testosterone and "age-related hypogonadism"–FDA concerns. N Engl J Med 2015;373(8):689–91.

67. Araujo AB, Esche GR, Kupelian V, et al. Prevalence of symptomatic androgen deficiency in men. J Clin Endocrinol Metab 2007;92(11):4241–7.

68. Wu FC, Tajar A, Beynon JM, et al. Identification of late-onset hypogonadism in middle-aged and elderly men. N Engl J Med 2010;363(2):123–35.

69. Orwoll E, Lambert LC, Marshall LM, et al. Testosterone and estradiol among older men. J Clin Endocrinol Metab 2006;91(4):1336–44.

70. Bhasin S, Pencina M, Jasuja GK, et al. Reference ranges for testosterone in men generated using liquid chromatography tandem mass spectrometry in a community-based sample of healthy nonobese young men in the Framingham Heart Study and applied to three geographically distinct cohorts. J Clin Endocrinol Metab 2011;96(8):2430–9.

71. Mohr BA, Bhasin S, Link CL, et al. The effect of changes in adiposity on testosterone levels in older men: longitudinal results from the Massachusetts Male Aging Study. Eur J Endocrinol 2006;155(3): 443–52.

72. Bhasin S, Jasuja GK, Pencina M, et al. Sex hormone-binding globulin, but not testosterone, is associated prospectively and independently with incident metabolic syndrome in men: the Framingham Heart Study. Diabetes Care 2011;34(11):2464–70.

73. Lakshman KM, Bhasin S, Araujo AB. Sex hormone-binding globulin as an independent predictor of incident type 2 diabetes mellitus in men. J Gerontol A Biol Sci Med Sci 2010;65(5):503–9.

74. Yialamas MA, Dwyer AA, Hanley E, et al. Acute sex steroid withdrawal reduces insulin sensitivity in healthy men with idiopathic hypogonadotropic hypogonadism. J Clin Endocrinol Metab 2007;92(11): 4254–9.

75. Basaria S, Muller DC, Carducci MA, et al. Relation between duration of androgen deprivation therapy and degree of insulin resistance in men with prostate cancer. Arch Intern Med 2007;167(6):612–3.

76. Woodhouse LJ, Gupta N, Bhasin M, et al. Dose-dependent effects of testosterone on regional adipose tissue distribution in healthy young men. J Clin Endocrinol Metab 2004;89(2):718–26.

77. Jones TH, Arver S, Behre HM, et al, TIMES2 Investigators. Testosterone replacement in hypogonadal men with type 2 diabetes and/or metabolic syndrome (the TIMES2 study). Diabetes Care 2011; 34(4):828–37.

78. Emmelot-Vonk MH, Verhaar HJ, Nakhai-Pour HR, et al. Low testosterone concentrations and the symptoms of testosterone deficiency according to the Androgen Deficiency in Ageing Males (ADAM) and Ageing Males' Symptoms rating scale (AMS) questionnaires. Clin Endocrinol (Oxf) 2011;74(4): 488–94.

79. Smith KW, Feldman HA, McKinlay JB. Construction and field validation of a self-administered screener for testosterone deficiency (hypogonadism) in ageing men. Clin Endocrinol (Oxf) 2000;53(6):703–11.

80. Veale D, Miles S, Bramley S, et al. Am I normal? A systematic review and construction of nomograms for flaccid and erect penis length and circumference in up to 15,521 men. BJU Int 2015;115(6):978–86.

81. Brambilla DJ, O'Donnell AB, Matsumoto AM, et al. Intraindividual variation in levels of serum testosterone and other reproductive and adrenal hormones in men. Clin Endocrinol (Oxf) 2007;67(6):853–62.

82. Bhasin S, Zhang A, Coviello A, et al. The impact of assay quality and reference ranges on clinical decision making in the diagnosis of androgen disorders. Steroids 2008;73(13):1311–7.

83. Ohlsson C, Lunetta KL, Stolk L, et al. Genetic determinants of serum testosterone concentrations in men. PLoS Genet 2011;7(10):e1002313.

84. Vermeulen A, Verdonck L, Kaufman JM. A critical evaluation of simple methods for the estimation of free testosterone in serum. J Clin Endocrinol Metab 1999;84(10):3666–72.

85. Zakharov MN, Bhasin S, Travison TG, et al. A multistep, dynamic allosteric model of testosterone's binding to sex hormone binding globulin. Mol Cell Endocrinol 2015;399:190–200.

86. Bhasin S, Basaria S. Diagnosis and treatment of hypogonadism in men. Best Pract Res Clin Endocrinol Metab 2011;25(2):251–70.

87. Cooper TG, Noonan E, Eckardstein SV, et al. World Health Organization reference values for human semen characteristics. Hum Reprod Update 2010;16(3):231–45.

Assays of Serum Testosterone

Amin S. Herati, MD[a], Cenk Cengiz, BS[a], Dolores J. Lamb, PhD[a,b,*]

KEYWORDS

- Adult • Humans • Testosterone/blood • Steroids/blood • Circadian rhythm
- Hypogonadism/metabolism • Testosterone/deficiency • Immunoassay

KEY POINTS

- Hypogonadism is increasing in prevalence as the population ages and obesity rates climb.
- The diagnosis of hypogonadism depends on an assessment of the clinical signs and symptoms of hypogonadism and the determination of serum testosterone levels.
- Significant variability can exist in serum total and free testosterone levels due to intraindividual variation and assay variability.
- Current serum testosterone assay methods include immunoassay and mass spectrometry. However, no current gold standard assay exists for the assessment of total testosterone levels.
- Standardization programs are in place to improve the accuracy and comparability of testosterone assays in clinical and research laboratories.

INTRODUCTION

Male hypogonadism is defined by the Endocrine Society as a clinical syndrome that results from the inability of the testes to produce physiologic levels of testosterone (T) and a "normal" number of spermatozoa secondary to a dysfunction in the hypothalamic-pituitary-gonadal axis (HPG).[1] The diagnosis of hypogonadism depends on the assessment of the clinical signs and symptoms of hypogonadism and serum T levels assayed on at least 2 different occasions.[2] The symptoms most suggestive are low libido followed by a reduced quality of erections; however, these markers are subjective and nonspecific.[3] The laboratory's assessment of serum T levels, in contrast, provides an objective measure of the gonadal status that can support or refute clinical signs and symptoms. Nevertheless, serum T levels can vary widely between samples drawn from the same patient and between the various laboratory assay platforms due to a multitude of factors, such as diurnal variation, systemic illnesses, and seasonal variation, as well as assay-specific factors, and must be interpreted with caution.

Current clinical laboratory assay platforms include immunoassays and mass spectrometry (MS). Despite significant advances to improve the accuracy and precision of currently available assays, limited comparability exists between assays at the lower and upper extremes of the T range. Moreover, there is no currently accepted gold standard method of assessment. In this review, the growing significance of T assays in the aging population is highlighted, the indications

Funding: A.S. Herati is a National Institutes of Health K12 Scholar supported by a Male Reproductive Health Research (MHRH) Career Development Physician-Scientist Award (HD073917-01) from the Eunice Kennedy Shriver National Institute of Child Health and Human Development Program (to D.J. Lamb).
[a] Scott Department of Urology, Center for Reproductive Medicine, Baylor College of Medicine, 1 Baylor Plaza, Houston, TX 77030, USA; [b] Department of Molecular and Cellular Biology, Baylor College of Medicine, 1 Baylor Plaza, Houston, TX 77030, USA
* Corresponding author. Scott Department of Urology, Center for Reproductive Medicine, Baylor College of Medicine, 1 Baylor Plaza, Suite N730, Houston, TX 77030.
E-mail address: dlamb@bcm.edu

for the various assays used to assess free and total T are discussed, and the impact of various preanalytical and analytical factors that can influence the results of T assays are analyzed.

PREVALENCE

Late-onset hypogonadism is considered to be a disease of aging. As the population ages, the epidemiologic burden of male hypogonadism is expected to proportionally increase. The World Health Organization estimates that by 2020, the number of people over the age of 65 will for the first time surpass the number of people less than 5 years of age.[4] According to the same estimates, the number of people over the age of 65 will nearly double from a current population of 524 million people to roughly 1.5 billion by 2050. A population-based observational study by Araujo and colleagues[5] estimated the crude prevalence of biochemically confirmed, symptomatic male hypogonadism (total T <300 ng/dL) to be 5.6% in a cohort of 1475 US men aged 30 to 79 and 18.4% in subset of men aged 70 to 79. The investigators projected in this study that in 2025, as many as 6.5 million American men will exhibit symptomatic androgen deficiency. In addition, comorbidities that accumulate as part of aging can also increase the epidemiologic burden of hypogonadism. The Healthy Man Study showed a strong association between comorbidities, such as obesity and ex-smoker status, and T values over repeat measures drawn over a 3-month duration.[6] Based on these trends, a significant increase in utilization of T assays can be expected, and a thorough understanding of the nuances and limitations of the various T assay platforms will be invaluable in the care of the hypogonadal patient.

DIAGNOSING HYPOGONADISM

Male hypogonadism results from a reduction of androgen levels due to a dysfunction in the HPG axis. The presence and magnitude of symptoms associated with male hypogonadism depend on the concentration of T available to the target organ. Although the total testosterone (TT) concentration is often used as a surrogate for the amount of T available for the target organ, the bioavailable fraction of the TT is a more accurate measure of T concentrations at the tissue level and correlates better with clinical symptoms than TT.[3,7,8] T circulates in either a protein-bound or non-protein-bound (free) state. In a healthy adult man, most T circulates in a protein-bound state attached to either albumin ~50%, sex hormone-binding globulin (SHBG) ~44%, or cortisol-binding globulin

~3.5%. The remaining 2% to 3% of T circulates as unbound, free testosterone (FT).[9,10] The bioavailable fraction of the TT consists of albumin-bound and FT. Unlike the TT level, the bioavailable fraction is not susceptible to SHBG concentration, which can fluctuate with age, thyroid function, drugs and alcohol consumption, and disorders of the pituitary and the liver.[11]

Diagnosing hypogonadism is challenging in the setting of a patient with the signs and symptoms consistent with hypogonadism, borderline normal TT value, and possible alteration of SHBG level. Under these circumstances, the Endocrine Society recommends measuring free or bioavailable testosterone (BioT) levels with an accurate and reliable assay.[1] Several methods have been used to assess FT and BioT levels, such as equilibrium dialysis (FT_D),[12] direct estimation of serum free T by an analogue ligand immunoassay (FT_A),[13] ammonium sulfate precipitation of SHBG-bound T,[14] calculation of the free androgen index (FAI) using the formula TT/(SHBG × 100),[15] and multiple algorithms to calculate the free testosterone index (FTI) based on the concentration of albumin and SHBG. Although the FT_D is considered the gold standard, this method is time-consuming and expensive.[16] In contrast, calculation of the FTI using published algorithms, such as the Vermeulen equation,[17] is inexpensive and has been shown to have good correlation with gold standard methods of comparison.[17–22]

The Vermeulen equation, which is widely used, determines the FT level using the concentration of T bound to albumin and the albumin concentration.[17] The equation operates under the assumption that the albumin concentration is in the physiologic range of 40 to 50 g/L (5.8–7.2 × 10^{-4} mol/L).[17] There are several shortcomings to this equation. If the albumin concentration is expected to deviate from the physiologic range, Vermeulen and colleagues[17] recommend calculating the albumin concentration in order to account for the reduced amount of albumin-bound T. In addition, the Vermeulen equation assumes that T does not face significant competition from other steroid hormones, such as estradiol (E2) and dihydrotestosterone (DHT), for its binding site on albumin.[16] Supraphysiologic levels of E2 and DHT will confound the calculation, leading to underestimation of the FT.

In a cross-sectional study of 50 men aged 28 to 90, Morley and colleagues[22] compared the results of different tissue-available T assays, including the ammonium sulfate precipitation method, FT_D, FT by ultracentrifugation (FT_U), FT_A, FTI, and TT, to determine the utility of each assay in the assessment of gonadal status. The investigators compared the week-to-week variability in BioT and TT levels in a subcohort of 16 men with a mean age of 69.3 ± 1.7 years. The investigators also compared the various assays to FT_D, with the best correlation being with FTI (r = 0.807) followed by BioT levels determined using ammonium sulfate precipitation (r = 0.670). When hypogonadism was defined as a TT value of 300 ng/dL or less and compared with BioT levels derived from the ammonium sulfate precipitation assay, 26% of men deemed eugonadal based on TT values were subsequently classified as hypogonadal based on the BioT values, whereas 16% of men classified as hypogonadal using TT values were reassessed as eugonadal based on BioT values. Morley and colleagues[22] also showed considerable variability in both TT and BioT levels over an 8-week period in a subgroup of 16 men.

In men with signs and symptoms of hypogonadism and no suspected alterations in the SHBG level, the TT level has sufficient sensitivity to diagnose hypogonadism. Morris and colleagues[20] demonstrated this in a cross-sectional study of 1072 men who were undergoing coronary angiography. TT, SHBG, and BioT levels (using ammonium sulfate precipitation) were measured, and FAI and FTI levels were calculated. Of the assessed methods, TT was the best predictor of BioT levels in the whole cohort, whereas SHBG and FAI values were the worst predictors of BioT levels. However, when the serum assay methods were assessed for their power to diagnose hypogonadism using the area under the receiver operating curve values, calculated free T outperformed TT (0.75 vs 0.63) in the subgroup of men with an TT greater than 7.5 nmol/L but less than 12 nmol/L. The Endocrine Society Clinical Practice Guidelines, therefore, recommends measuring the morning TT value as an initial diagnostic test and the bioavailable T level in men with low normal TT values.[1]

REFERENCE RANGES OF TESTOSTERONE

Despite the increasing use of T assays in research and clinical practice, no universally accepted cutoff value exists for hypogonadism.[23] Although TT values less than 200 ng/dL are considered diagnostic for hypogonadism, levels between 200 and 320 ng/dL are considered equivocal because of the variable presence of symptoms at different cutoff values in different patients and the lack of agreement among the platform assays used.[24,25] Several preanalytical and analytical factors can alter the specificity and precision of an assay, including technical limitations of the assay and intraindividual variation. This variation is major problem because different assays and laboratories lack

comparability in results, especially with lower T values.[25,26]

In order to address the lack of comparability, the Endocrine Society along with the Centers for Disease Control and Prevention (CDC), National Center for Environmental Health, and Division of Laboratory Sciences have set forth an external quality control program called the CDC Laboratory/Manufacturer Hormone Standardization (CDC HoSt) program to reduce the measurement bias and improve the comparability of T testing methods.[25–27] The CDC HoSt program provides common calibrators derived from individual donor sera with known target values to align the assay results of participating laboratories. Four sets of 10 serum samples with undisclosed T concentrations are sent to the participating laboratories for analysis of accuracy and performance evaluation. Between 2007 and 2011, utilization of the HoSt program reduced the measurement bias observed among mass spectrometric (MS) methods by approximately 50%.[28]

VARIATION IN TESTOSTERONE

Differences in TT and FT levels can be due to intraindividual and assay variability. Intraindividual variation, which can be caused by circadian rhythmicity, has a more profound effect on variability.[29]

INTRAINDIVIDUAL VARIATION

Both TT and FT exhibit circadian rhythmicity with peaks in the morning and troughs in the evening.[30] This diurnal variation of total and free T is most pronounced in young men and is blunted with increasing age.[31–33] In a study comparing a cohort of 18 young men (age 21–37 years) to 28 elderly men (age 67–98 year), morning plasma T levels were 33% higher than evening T levels in the younger cohort (P<.01), but only 8.4% higher in the older cohort (P>.05).[34] This circadian rhythmicity was also observed by Diver and colleagues,[33] who performed sequential measurements of TT, FT, BioT, and SHBG every 30 minutes for 24 hours in 10 healthy, young men aged 23 to 33 years and 8 healthy men aged 55 to 64 years. Statistically significant variation was seen in all 4 indices of androgen status with a minimum of 43% reduction seen in TT from peak levels observed between 06.00h and 10.00h to nadir levels seen between 18.00h and 22.00h in both the young and middle-aged groups. Although more recent data published by Welliver and colleagues[35] showed in a population of men presenting for erectile dysfunction that the difference between TT levels were statistically significant between 7.00h and 9.00h and 9.00h and 14.00h in men younger than 45 years of age. This difference, however, was not statistically significant in men over the age of 45. The investigators recommended assessing T levels in men younger than 45 as close to 7.00h as possible and before 14.00h in men older than 45 years of age. These findings were corroborated by Crawford and colleagues,[36] who more recently showed no significant difference in TT values drawn between 8.00h and 11.0h, 11.00h and 14.00h, and 20.00h to 8.00h in a population of elderly men with a mean age of 61. The current recommendation of the International Society of Andrology, the International Society for Study of the Aging Male, the European Association of Urology, the European Association of Andrology, and the American Society of Andrology, however, remains for a serum TT level to be obtained between 07.00h and 11.00h.[37]

Moreover, T values can fluctuate from day to day and week to week within the same individual. A study of aging men between 55 and 70 years found TT to vary by 14.8% (range 0.1%–79%) when values were reassessed on 2 different days within the same month.[38] Morley and colleagues[22] showed significant variability of both TT and BioT levels over a course of 8 weeks. Over this course, 8 of 16 men who were eugonadal at one time point were hypogonadal at a second time point. Vermeulen and Verdonck[39] showed a similar degree of variability in a cohort of 169 men aged 40 to 80 with symptomatic benign prostatic hyperplasia observed with 8 serum T level checks over a 50-week period. Although good correlation was observed (r = 0.849) between the first sampling and the 7 subsequent samples, the mean coefficient of variation (CV) was 16.9% ± 8.4% with 9 men demonstrating greater than 25% variation. Some of this variation can be attributed to biological influences, such as heat exposure, physical training, alcohol withdrawal, and medications.[40] Acute and subacute illnesses can also introduce significant variation in T levels; therefore, the Endocrine Society has recommended delaying the evaluation of androgen deficiency until the illness has resolved.[1]

Reportedly, laboratory errors occur in 0.6% of inpatient and 0.04% of outpatient laboratory tests and can introduce significant heterogeneity in assay results.[41] The vast majority of laboratory errors occur in the preanalytical phase with a frequency as high as 84.5%.[26,42] Common errors that can occur in this phase are incorrect patient identification/mislabeling, inappropriate container/ tube used, inappropriate storage or transfer, or inappropriate quantity or quality of specimen.[42] In a systematic review of errors in laboratory medicine, Bonini and colleagues[41] found the highest rate of outpatient laboratory errors was attributable to incorrect labeling of the sample (36.4%) followed by hemolysis of the sample (32.3%). The investigators recommend routine auditing of rejected samples to determine what factors are associated with rejected samples. Centrifuging a sample of blood and delaying its analysis can cause an underestimation of TT values.[40] Attention must also be paid to the temperature of the sample, not to allow it to reach room temperature. In contrast, TT and BioT levels can be determined from serum stored at -70°C for up to 7 years with excellent stability.[22] Other important preanalytical factors to consider are the type of blood collection tube and the properties of the collection tube, including whether it is glass versus plastic. Additives, such as clot activators, can cause a 4-fold increase in TT, and anticoagulant additives, such as EDTA and sodium citrate, can alter SHBG levels and impair FT level determination.[40,43,44] Attention must be paid to the above factors in order to minimize the amount of laboratory error introduced and prevent unintended clinical consequences of a spurious laboratory value.

METHODS FOR MEASURING TOTAL TESTOSTERONE
Immunoassays

Immunoassays are widely used in the clinical laboratory to measure TT levels. The 2 most frequently used assays are radioimmunoassay (RIA) and chemiluminescent immunoassays, both of which can be performed directly on serum or plasma after extraction and/or chromatography.[25] The additional extraction and chromatography step, although more labor-intensive, removes interfering proteins and cross-reacting hormones. RIAs measure T by incubating patient serum with anti-T antibodies bound to radioactive antigen. As the antigen within the patient serum dislodges the radioactive antigen from the antigen-binding site, the particles released can be measured to identify total androgen concentration. Chemiluminescent assays, however, have a secondary component, which is an antibody bound to an enzyme, commonly horseradish peroxidase. T can be measured by incubating patient serum in one well coated with antibody specific to the hormone. The secondary antibody is then added to this complex followed by a chemiluminescent substrate. The antibody-conjugated enzyme digests this substrate in a reaction producing a detectable luminescent signal. The absorbance of the signal can be read using a spectrophotometer, and the antigen concentration can be calculated by making use of known standards run on the same plate.

Clinical immunoassays for hormone measurement can be technically simple, rapid, and relatively affordable.[25] With each additional run conducted on a high-speed automated platform or even using a single 96-well plate, cost-effectiveness and turnaround time improve, thereby creating a high throughput. Although immunoassays can be very useful, they do have drawbacks. T concentrations may be overestimated and are vulnerable to matrix effects.[45] Moreover, accuracy is limited for T levels less than 300 ng/dL when performed without extraction and chromatographic steps, and differences between reference intervals in different populations are not well documented in scientific literature.[22,23,46,47] In addition, RIA, which is rarely if ever used in today's clinical diagnostic laboratories, also carries the disadvantage of creating radioactive waste. Importantly, because these assays use antibodies targeting specific chemical moieties on the steroid molecules and show high specificity for T or DHT, they will not detect anabolic steroids lacking this structure. Accordingly, an anabolic steroid user will show low levels of circulating T measured by immunoassay, despite appearing highly masculinized.

Several studies reported acceptable agreement among immunoassays for determining T concentrations characteristic of healthy, eugonadal men but poor reliability and agreement in detecting low to very low T concentrations characteristic of hypogonadal men, women, and children. In a comparison of 10 immunoassay platforms against the reference method isotope-dilution gas chromatography-mass spectrometry (ID/GC-MS), Taieb and colleagues[48] showed significant overestimation of the immunoassay platforms below a concentration of 80 nmol/L. Seven of the 10 immunoassays overestimated the T values with up to a 5-fold difference in values observed with the Immulite 2000 platform (Siemens Medical Solutions Diagnostics, Los Angeles, CA) compared with ID/GC-MS. Similar findings were observed by Wang and colleagues,[49] who compared 6 immunoassays to liquid chromatography (LC)/MS-MS. Despite a high intraclass correlation (range 0.92–0.97) among the immunoassays, a lack of precision and accuracy was present at low serum T concentrations (<100 ng/dL). Further supporting this finding was a subsequent study by Moal and colleagues,[50] who compared 5 immunoassays to LC-MS/MS in a population of 70 women and children. The investigators found poor reliability of the immunoassays at low serum T concentrations with all assays overestimating the T levels.

Mass Spectrometry

In order to address the shortcomings in the specificity and precision of the immunoassays, particularly at low to very-low levels of T, MS with chromatography has increasingly transitioned from a laboratory research technique to clinical application because of its capability of detecting multiple analytes in a single run, accuracy over a wide range of concentrations, specificity to detect the compound of interest, and immunity to error from antibody cross-reactivity.[51,52] MS involves sample preparation to remove interfering matrix (such as salts, proteins, and phospholipids), chromatographic separation, ionization of the analyte, and analysis with a spectrometer.[52,53] Chromatographic separation can be performed in a gas phase (GC) or a liquid phase (LC). LC is preferred over GC for blood specimens because LC requires lower specimen volume, is less time consuming, is more amenable to automation, and does not require chemical steroid derivatization.[51,53] In contrast, GC provides a more comprehensive screen of an individual's steroid profile, which is particularly useful in the clinical setting of an athlete or body builder who is using an anabolic-androgenic steroid and has a profoundly low T level.[51] The specificity and accuracy of MS have also increased by the performance of tandem (MS/MS) by applying a second round of ionization to further fragment the analyte ions of interest to improve the discriminant ability of the assay. The heightened sensitivity and specificity of LC-MS/MS have allowed for the quantification of free, unbound T in saliva with enough sensitivity to detect as little as 5 pmol/L of T in the female saliva.[54] However, MS is not available in all laboratories because of the requirement of high technical expertise, high operating cost, lack of standardization, and use of solvents that require special disposal.[25,52]

In order to determine the precision and limits of quantification (LOQ) of the available MS methods, several studies have compared the different MS methods to each other. Thienpont and colleagues[55] compared 58 samples obtained from 40 men and 10 women using 5 different ID-MS measurement procedures, including 4 different ID-LC-MS/MS assays and 1 ID-GC-MS assay. For T concentrations greater than 5 nmol/L, minimal variation was seen between the assays with a CV value range of 2.0% to 6.6%. Slightly higher variation and less precision were seen in the less than 5 nmol/L range with a CV range of 3.9% to 8.5%. These assays were able to detect very low T concentrations with LOQ values ranging from 0.035 to 0.3 nmol/L for all 5 assays. In a similar experiment, Vesper and colleagues[56] compared sera obtained from 12 women and 8 men using 7 different LC-MS/MS assays and 1 GC-MS assay. The between-laboratory variability for all 8 assays increased with smaller T concentrations with less than 15% CV for concentrations greater than 1.53 nmol/L compared with less than 34% at 0.3 nmol/L. Within-run variability was also assessed using 5 replicate samples obtained from both a male and a female subject. Greater variability was again seen at lower T concentrations with a CV range of 1.4% to 11.36% for a T concentration of 10.3 nmol/L versus a wider CV range of 2.5% to 25.6% for a T level of 0.29 nmol/L. A newer method of MS called high-turbulence flow LC and atmospheric pressure chemical ionization-MS/MS has been described with narrower CV values (7.6%–10.8% for intra-assay and 9.8%–13.4% for interassay) and lower LOQ (0.3 ng/dL); however, data are lacking on its comparison to other established MS methods.

The precision and accuracy of the MS have been attributed to the degree of preparation of the analyte before performing MS and the calibration of the assay. One important factor that can influence the accuracy of the assay is the presence of nonvolatile compounds (such as salts, drugs/metabolites, and endogenous compounds), which can influence the efficiency of sample vaporization and result in less analyte reaching the detector in the mass spectrometer. This factor, however, can be controlled for with calibration and the use of internal standards. MS standardization through the use of common calibrators is a focus of the CDC HoSt program to reduce the variability among MS assays.[27]

SUMMARY

The diagnosis of male hypogonadism is as much based on the clinical findings as it is on the laboratory results. When considering T levels, consideration must be given to the preanalytical and analytical factors that may be influencing the levels in every clinical circumstance. Although there is no current gold standard assay for the assessment of TT levels, every laboratory should establish reference ranges for their patient population. The standardization of immunoassays and MS assays through external quality control programs, such as the CDC HoSt program, will not only improve the accuracy and the interpretability of assay results for clinical and research purposes but also facilitate public health activities.

REFERENCES

1. Bhasin S, Cunningham GR, Hayes FJ, et al. Testosterone therapy in men with androgen deficiency syndromes: an Endocrine Society clinical practice guideline. J Clin Endocrinol Metab 2010;95(6): 2536–59.
2. Quigley CA, De Bellis A, Marschke KB, et al. Androgen receptor defects: historical, clinical, and molecular perspectives. Endocr Rev 1995;16(3): 271–321.
3. Morley JE, Charlton E, Patrick P, et al. Validation of a screening questionnaire for androgen deficiency in aging males. Metabolism 2000;49(9):1239–42.
4. Wolrd Health Organization. Global health and aging. 2011. Available at: https://d2cauhfh6h4x0p.cloudfront. net/s3fs-public/global_health_and_aging.pdf. Accessed November 28, 2015.
5. Araujo AB, Esche GR, Kupelian V, et al. Prevalence of symptomatic androgen deficiency in men. J Clin Endocrinol Metab 2007;92(11):4241–7.
6. Sartorius G, Spasevska S, Idan A, et al. Serum testosterone, dihydrotestosterone and estradiol concentrations in older men self-reporting very good health: the healthy man study. Clin Endocrinol (Oxf) 2012;77(5):755–63.
7. Nankin HR, Calkins JH. Decreased bioavailable testosterone in aging normal and impotent men. J Clin Endocrinol Metab 1986;63(6):1418–20.
8. Morley JE, Kaiser F, Raum WJ, et al. Potentially predictive and manipulable blood serum correlates of aging in the healthy human male: progressive decreases in bioavailable testosterone, dehydroepiandrosterone sulfate, and the ratio of insulin-like growth factor 1 to growth hormone. Proc Natl Acad Sci U S A 1997;94(14):7537–42.
9. Diver MJ. Laboratory measurement of testosterone. Front Horm Res 2009;37:21–31.
10. Dunn JF, Nisula BC, Rodbard D. Transport of steroid hormones: binding of 21 endogenous steroids to both testosterone-binding globulin and corticosteroid-binding globulin in human plasma. J Clin Endocrinol Metab 1981;53(1):58–68.
11. Thaler MA, Seifert-Klauss V, Luppa PB. The biomarker sex hormone-binding globulin—from established applications to emerging trends in clinical medicine. Best Pract Res Clin Endocrinol Metab 2015;29(5):749–60.
12. Miller KK, Rosner W, Lee H, et al. Measurement of free testosterone in normal women and women with androgen deficiency: comparison of methods. J Clin Endocrinol Metab 2004;89(2):525–33.
13. Van Uytfanghe K, Stockl D, Kaufman JM, et al. Validation of 5 routine assays for serum free testosterone with a candidate reference measurement procedure based on ultrafiltration and isotope dilution-gas chromatography-mass spectrometry. Clin Biochem 2005;38(3):253–61.
14. Tremblay RR, Dube JY. Plasma concentrations of free and non-TeBG bound testosterone in women on oral contraceptives. Contraception 1974;10(6): 599–605.

15. Wilke TJ, Utley DJ. Total testosterone, free-androgen index, calculated free testosterone, and free testosterone by analog RIA compared in hirsute women and in otherwise-normal women with altered binding of sex-hormone-binding globulin. Clin Chem 1987; 33(8):1372–5.

16. de Ronde W, van der Schouw YT, Pols HA, et al. Calculation of bioavailable and free testosterone in men: a comparison of 5 published algorithms. Clin Chem 2006;52(9):1777–84.

17. Vermeulen A, Verdonck L, Kaufman JM. A critical evaluation of simple methods for the estimation of free testosterone in serum. J Clin Endocrinol Metab 1999;84(10):3666–72.

18. Sodergard R, Backstrom T, Shanbhag V, et al. Calculation of free and bound fractions of testosterone and estradiol-17 beta to human plasma proteins at body temperature. J Steroid Biochem 1982;16(6):801–10.

19. Emadi-Konjin P, Bain J, Bromberg IL. Evaluation of an algorithm for calculation of serum "bioavailable" testosterone (BAT). Clin Biochem 2003;36(8):591–6.

20. Morris PD, Malkin CJ, Channer KS, et al. A mathematical comparison of techniques to predict biologically available testosterone in a cohort of 1072 men. Eur J Endocrinol 2004;151(2):241–9.

21. Ly LP, Handelsman DJ. Empirical estimation of free testosterone from testosterone and sex hormone-binding globulin immunoassays. Eur J Endocrinol 2005;152(3):471–8.

22. Morley JE, Patrick P, Perry HM 3rd. Evaluation of assays available to measure free testosterone. Metabolism 2002;51(5):554–9.

23. Paduch DA, Brannigan RE, Fuchs EF, et al. The laboratory diagnosis of testosterone deficiency. Urology 2014;83(5):980–8.

24. Vermeulen A. Hormonal cut-offs of partial androgen deficiency: a survey of androgen assays. J Endocrinol Invest 2005;28(3 Suppl):28–31.

25. Rosner W, Auchus RJ, Azziz R, et al. Position statement: utility, limitations, and pitfalls in measuring testosterone: an Endocrine Society position statement. J Clin Endocrinol Metab 2007;92(2):405–13.

26. Vesper HW, Botelho JC, Shacklady C, et al. CDC project on standardizing steroid hormone measurements. Steroids 2008;73(13):1286–92.

27. Rosner W, Vesper H. Preface. CDC workshop report improving steroid hormone measurements in patient care and research translation. Steroids 2008;73(13): 1285.

28. Vesper HW, Botelho JC, Wang Y. Challenges and improvements in testosterone and estradiol testing. Asian J Androl 2014;16(2):178–84.

29. Brambilla DJ, O'Donnell AB, Matsumoto AM, et al. Intraindividual variation in levels of serum testosterone and other reproductive and adrenal hormones in men. Clin Endocrinol (Oxf) 2007;67(6):853–62.

30. Tenover JS, Matsumoto AM, Clifton DK, et al. Age-related alterations in the circadian rhythms of pulsatile luteinizing hormone and testosterone secretion in healthy men. J Gerontol 1988;43(6): M163–9.

31. Plymate SR, Tenover JS, Bremner WJ. Circadian variation in testosterone, sex hormone-binding globulin, and calculated non-sex hormone-binding globulin bound testosterone in healthy young and elderly men. J Androl 1989;10(5):366–71.

32. Bremner WJ, Vitiello MV, Prinz PN. Loss of circadian rhythmicity in blood testosterone levels with aging in normal men. J Clin Endocrinol Metab 1983;56(6): 1278–81.

33. Diver MJ, Imtiaz KE, Ahmad AM, et al. Diurnal rhythms of serum total, free and bioavailable testosterone and of SHBG in middle-aged men compared with those in young men. Clin Endocrinol (Oxf) 2003; 58(6):710–7.

34. Marrama P, Carani C, Baraghini GF, et al. Circadian rhythm of testosterone and prolactin in the ageing. Maturitas 1982;4(2):131–8.

35. Welliver RC Jr, Wiser HJ, Brannigan RE, et al. Validity of midday total testosterone levels in older men with erectile dysfunction. J Urol 2014;192(1): 165–9.

36. Crawford ED, Poage W, Nyhuis A, et al. Measurement of testosterone: how important is a morning blood draw? Curr Med Res Opin 2015;31(10): 1911–4.

37. Wang C, Nieschlag E, Swerdloff R, et al. Investigation, treatment, and monitoring of late-onset hypogonadism in males: ISA, ISSAM, EAU, EAA, and ASA recommendations. J Androl 2009;30(1):1–9.

38. Christ-Crain M, Meier C, Huber P, et al. Comparison of different methods for the measurement of serum testosterone in the aging male. Swiss Med Wkly 2004;134(13–14):193–7.

39. Vermeulen A, Verdonck G. Representativeness of a single point plasma testosterone level for the long term hormonal milieu in men. J Clin Endocrinol Metab 1992;74(4):939–42.

40. Raff H, Sluss PM. Pre-analytical issues for testosterone and estradiol assays. Steroids 2008;73(13): 1297–304.

41. Bonini P, Plebani M, Ceriotti F, et al. Errors in laboratory medicine. Clin Chem 2002;48(5):691–8.

42. Wiwanitkit V. Types and frequency of preanalytical mistakes in the first Thai ISO 9002:1994 certified clinical laboratory, a 6-month monitoring. BMC Clin Pathol 2001;1(1):5.

43. Kohek M, Leme C, Nakamura IT, et al. Effects of EDTA and sodium citrate on hormone measurements by fluorometric (FIA) and immunofluorometric (IFMA) methods. BMC Clin Pathol 2002;2(1):2.

44. Wang C, Shiraishi S, Leung A, et al. Validation of a testosterone and dihydrotestosterone liquid

chromatography tandem mass spectrometry assay: Interference and comparison with established methods. Steroids 2008;73(13):1345–52.

45. Elder PA, Lewis JG. An enzyme-linked immunosorbent assay (ELISA) for plasma testosterone. J Steroid Biochem 1985;22(5):635–8.

46. Matsumoto AM, Bremner WJ. Serum testosterone assays–accuracy matters. J Clin Endocrinol Metab 2004;89(2):520–4.

47. Fuqua JS, Sher ES, Migeon CJ, et al. Assay of plasma testosterone during the first six months of life: importance of chromatographic purification of steroids. Clin Chem 1995;41(8 Pt 1):1146–9.

48. Taieb J, Mathian B, Millot F, et al. Testosterone measured by 10 immunoassays and by isotope-dilution gas chromatography-mass spectrometry in sera from 116 men, women, and children. Clin Chem 2003;49(8):1381–95.

49. Wang C, Catlin DH, Demers LM, et al. Measurement of total serum testosterone in adult men: comparison of current laboratory methods versus liquid chromatography-tandem mass spectrometry. J Clin Endocrinol Metab 2004;89(2):534–43.

50. Moal V, Mathieu E, Reynier P, et al. Low serum testosterone assayed by liquid chromatography-tandem mass spectrometry. Comparison with five immunoassay techniques. Clin Chim Acta 2007; 386(1–2):12–9.

51. Krone N, Hughes BA, Lavery GG, et al. Gas chromatography/mass spectrometry (GC/MS) remains a pre-eminent discovery tool in clinical steroid investigations even in the era of fast liquid chromatography tandem mass spectrometry (LC/MS/MS). J Steroid Biochem Mol Biol 2010;121(3–5):496–504.

52. Stanczyk FZ, Clarke NJ. Advantages and challenges of mass spectrometry assays for steroid hormones. J Steroid Biochem Mol Biol 2010;121(3–5):491–5.

53. Strathmann FG, Hoofnagle AN. Current and future applications of mass spectrometry to the clinical laboratory. Am J Clin Pathol 2011;136(4):609–16.

54. Keevil BG, MacDonald P, Macdowall W, et al. Salivary testosterone measurement by liquid chromatography tandem mass spectrometry in adult males and females. Ann Clin Biochem 2014;51(Pt 3):368–78.

55. Thienpont LM, van Uytfanghe K, Blincko S, et al. State-of-the-art of serum testosterone measurement by isotope dilution-liquid chromatography-tandem mass spectrometry. Clin Chem 2008;54(8):1290–7.

56. Vesper HW, Bhasin S, Wang C, et al. Interlaboratory comparison study of serum total testosterone [corrected] measurements performed by mass spectrometry methods. Steroids 2009;74(6):498–503.

Testosterone Therapies

Mohit Khera, MD, MBA, MPH

KEYWORDS

• Testosterone • Therapies • Formulations • Gels • Androgens

KEY POINTS

- There are numerous testosterone formulations now available, and patients and clinicians should take into account the "4 Cs": cost, compliance, convenience, and concentration levels.
- Testosterone is a natural contraceptive and should not be used in men trying to achieve a pregnancy.
- All testosterone gels and solutions have an increased risk of transference, and there should be increased caution when in contact with children and pregnant women.

INTRODUCTION

Over the past decade, there has been exponential growth in sales of testosterone therapies and their utilization. In 2012, testosterone was one of the fastest growing medications in the United States. Much of the increased sales and utilization of testosterone can be attributed to an aging US population, decreased concern that testosterone can cause prostate cancer, increased awareness of the beneficial effects of testosterone, and direct to consumer advertising and marketing. There has been expansive growth in "testosterone centers" throughout the United States, signifying an increase in patient demand to seek treatment for this condition. Although in 2006 there were only 2 topical gels in the testosterone market, just a decade later there are now 6 topical formulations, new long-acting testosterone pellets and injections, and promising oral formulations on the horizon. Although there are many testosterone therapies available, patients and clinicians must decide the optimal formulation specifically for each patient.

HISTORY

The beneficial effects of testosterone have been known for thousands of years. Throughout history, numerous attempts have been made to use testosterone extracts to treat sexual dysfunction and reverse the aging process.[1] For example, in 2000 BC, the ancient Indian manuscripts described the ingestion of testicular tissue for the treatment of erectile dysfunction. The ancient Egyptians also described the medicinal powers of the testis. In 1889, a prominent French physiologist, Charles Brown-Sequard, injected himself with an extract of crushed canine and guinea pig testes and reported improvements in his urinary stream, intellect, and erectile function. Testicular transplants first began in 1912. In 1920, Serge Vornoff completed the first testicular tissue transplant from chimpanzee to human.[2] Testosterone therapy (TTh) officially started in 1935 when Enrest Lacquer isolated testosterone from bull testes, and in 1939 when Butenandt and Ruzicka first described the synthesis of testosterone. In the 1940s, the first subdermal testosterone implants were introduced, and 10 years later was the development of the first testosterone esters. These esters are the basis of the intramuscular (IM) injections that are used today. In the 1970s, testosterone undecanoate (TU; Andriol Testocaps, Organon) became available outside the United States. Currently, TU has recently been made available in the United States as a long-acting testosterone injection formulation. In 1994, the first transdermal testosterone was introduced as a patch, known as Testoderm (Alza Corporation), and in 2000, the first topical testosterone gel became available. Finally, in 2008, subdermal

Baylor College of Medicine, 7200 Cambridge Street, 10th Floor, Houston, TX 77030, USA
E-mail address: mkhera@bcm.edu

Urol Clin N Am 43 (2016) 185–193
http://dx.doi.org/10.1016/j.ucl.2016.01.004
0094-0143/16/$ – see front matter © 2016 Elsevier Inc. All rights reserved.

testosterone implants, and in 2014, nasal testosterone gels were the first to be US Food and Drug Administration (FDA) approved.

PRETREATMENT CONSIDERATIONS

In March 2015, the FDA issued a drug safety communication cautioning about the use of testosterone products for low testosterone due to aging. The manufacturers of testosterone products were also required by the FDA to amend the drug labels to also include warnings for possible increased risk of myocardial infarction and stroke. Revisions to all the testosterone labeling were completed in May 2015 and now include the following[3]:

Testosterone is indicated for replacement therapy in adult men for conditions associated with a deficiency or absence of endogenous testosterone.

Primary hypogonadism (congenital or acquired): testicular failure due to conditions such as crypotorchidism, bilateral torsion, orchitis, vanishing testis syndrome, orchiectomy, Klinefelter syndrome, chemotherapy, or toxic damage from alcohol or heavy metals. These men usually have low serum testosterone concentrations and gonadotropins (follicle-stimulating hormone, FSH; luteinizing hormone, LH) higher than the normal range.

Hypogonadotropic hypogonadism (congenital or acquired): gonadotropin or LH-releasing hormone deficiency or pituitary-hypothalamic injury from tumors, trauma, or radiation. These men have low testosterone serum concentrations, but gonadotropins in the normal or low range.

Safety and efficacy of testosterone in men with "age-related hypogonadism" (also referred to as "late-onset hypogonadism") have not been established.

Epidemiologic studies and randomized controlled trials have been inconclusive for determining the risk of major adverse cardiovascular events (MACE), such as nonfatal myocardial infarction, nonfatal stroke, and cardiovascular deaths, with the use of testosterone compared with nonuse. Some after-marketing studies, but not all, have reported increased risk of MACE in association with use of testosterone replacement therapy in men.

Before initiating TTh, several factors have to be taken into consideration. The "4 Cs" can help clinicians and patients determine which formation is most suitable. The "4 Cs" include cost, compliance, convenience, and concentration. Cost has become a major barrier for many patients trying to obtain access to TTh because many insurance carriers now have much more stringent criteria for which patients can receive coverage for TTh. A concern for many of the topical agents is their ability to penetrate the skin and obtain therapeutic serum testosterone levels. Not all gels are equally effective in all men, and at times, patients are required to switch to a different gel that may offer better serum testosterone concentration levels.[4] Some patients are not compliant with daily applications of testosterone, and in these patients, a long-acting testosterone formulation may be more appropriate. Other considerations before initiating TTh are the risk of transference and concerns for future fertility. Exogenous testosterone is a natural contraceptive and thus should not be used in men trying to achieve a pregnancy. In these men, methods to increase endogenous testosterone should be implored.

CONTRAINDICATIONS TO TESTOSTERONE THERAPY

The 2010 American Endocrine Guidelines state that TTh is contraindicated in patients with the following conditions[5]:

- Metastatic prostate cancer
- Breast cancer
- Unevaluated prostate nodule or induration
- Prostate-specific antigen (PSA) >4 ng/mL (>3 ng/mL in high-risk individuals)
- Hematocrit >50%
- Severe lower urinary tract symptoms associated with benign prostatic hypertrophy (BPH) as indicated by American Urological Association/International Prostate Symptom Score (IPSS) score >19
- Uncontrolled or poorly controlled congestive heart failure

The Endocrine Society recommends Urologic consultation for patients with a prostate nodule, elevated PSA greater than 4 ng/mL (>3 ng/mL in high-risk individuals), and IPSS scores greater than 19 before starting TTh. Urologists should use their own judgment in assessing prostate cancer and BPH risk on the basis of their clinical experience because TTh can be safely initiated in many of these patients if they are monitored carefully.

TREATMENT OPTIONS

Currently, most TTh users in the United States are receiving some form of transdermal gel therapy. In

2006, roughly 70% of the TTh users were using transdermal gel therapy; 17% were using testosterone injections; 10% were using transdermal testosterone patches; and 3% were using some other form of testosterone supplementation, such as an oral formulation. Options for transdermal androgen replacement include adhesive skin patches or gel applications. **Table 1** lists all available testosterone preparations and their characteristics.

TESTOSTERONE GELS AND SOLUTIONS

The stratum corneum of the skin serves as a reservoir for the testosterone, allowing its slow release over several hours.[6] Only 10% of the gels are absorbed in the skin, and thus, the remaining testosterone gel is at increased risk for transference. Currently, all testosterone liquids and gels in the United States contain an FDA black box warning for the risk of transference. Thus, the gel or liquid must be washed off before there is any skin-to-skin contact between the testosterone application site and another person. Patients using a testosterone gel or solution may experience higher levels of dihydrotestosterone (DHT) because the dermis contains 5-αreductase, which is responsible for converting testosterone into DHT.

Androgel 1% was the first topical testosterone gel available in June 2000. It now comes in 2 different concentrations: the original 1% and the new 1.62%. There are some differences between these 2 gels. For example, the starting dose of Androgel 1% is 50 mg of testosterone versus 40.5 mg of testosterone in Androgel 1.62%.[7,8] The maximum doses of testosterone in Androgel 1% and 1.62% are 100 mg and 81 mg, respectively. A patient can swim or shower after 6 hours with Androgel 1% versus 2 hours with Androgel 1.62%. Finally, unlike Androgel 1%, Androgel 1.62% is not indicated to be applied to the abdomen. Adverse effects specific for Androgel include acne, headaches, emotional lability, nervousness, and gynecomastia.

Testim was the second gel approved by the FDA in 2003. Testim is a 1% gel in which each tube contains 50 mg of testosterone.[9] The starting dose is 1 tube, but some patients can be titrated to 2 tubes, or 100 mg of testosterone. Testim is to be applied on the shoulders and upper arms. Testim in several studies has been shown to have good skin penetration and serum testosterone levels[4,10]; this is primarily due to its emollient pentadectalactone, which is found also in many aftershaves and colognes. Patients can swim or shower 2 hours after applying Testim.

Fortesta was approved by the FDA in 2010. Fortesta is a 2% gel that contains oleic acid, which is a known penetration enhancer.[11] This gel is applied to the inner thighs, and the starting dose is 40 mg. Each pump is 10 mg, and a total of 2 pumps are placed on each inner thigh. The dose can be titrated to 70 mg. Patients can swim or shower after 2 hours. The greatest adverse event with Fortesta is that up to 16% of patients may develop a skin reaction. Fortesta has been reported to restore testosterone concentrations in 77% of men in a study, without risk of supraphysiologic testosterone concentrations.[12]

Axiron was approved by the FDA in 2010. Axiron is a 2% testosterone liquid, not a gel, and is considered a solution.[12] This liquid is placed under the axilla. The starting dose is 60 mg and can be titrated to 120 mg. Each pump contains 30 mg of testosterone. The patient should apply his deodorant first and then the testosterone. Adverse effects of Axiron include application site erythema and irritation in 7% to 8%. Other adverse events include headaches, erythrocytosis, diarrhea, and vomiting.

Vogelxo was released in the United States in 2014. The starting dose is 50 mg, and the maximum dose is 100 mg.[13] This formulation comes in packets, tubes, or a pump. The gel is applied on the shoulder and upper arms. The most common side effects noted were erythrocytosis and skin irritation.

Natesto was approved by the FDA in 2014. Natesto is the first intranasal testosterone. Each pump of Natesto delivers 5.5 mg of testosterone.[14] The recommend dose is 11 mg 3 times daily, reaching maximum serum levels within 40 minutes with half-life ranging from 10 to 100 minutes. The most common adverse reactions include increase in PSA, headache, and local intranasal symptoms.

BUCCAL FORMULATIONS

Striant is currently the only buccal formulation of testosterone available in the United States. It is applied every 12 hours to the buccal mucosa above the incisor tooth.[15] Each tablet is 30 mg of testosterone. Striant avoids first-pass hepatic metabolism by direct absorption through the buccal mucosa. This delivery system allows for rapid absorption of testosterone and reaches a peak level in 30 minutes.[16] The application site should be rotated to minimize local gum irritation, which occurs in up to 10% of patients. Gum irritation is typically manifested as edema, gingivitis, and blistering and inflammation. Alteration of taste has also been described in some patients.

Table 1
Characteristics of available testosterone preparations

Route	Formulation	Dosing	Pros	Cons
Transdermal gels	• AndroGel 1%/1.62 • Fortesta • Axiron • Testim • Vogelxo	40 mg–120 mg every day	• Rapid onset	• Cost • Skin irritation • Transference
Nasal	Natesto 5.5 mg/pump	11 mg 3 times a day	• Rapid onset • Decreased risk of transference	• Nasal irritation • 3 times a day dosing
Topical patches	Androderm 2 mg/patch and 4 mg/ patches	2–6 mg every day	• No transference • Ease to use	Skin irritation
Oral buccal	Striant 30 mg tablet	30 mg 2 times a day	• Rapid onset • Easy to use	• Gum/mouth irritation • Inconvenient dosing
Short-acting injection	• Enanthate 200 mg/mL • Cypionate 100 or 200 mg/mL	100 mg IM every q week or 200 mg every 2 wk	• Cost • Improved compliance	• Fluctuating testosterone levels • Testosterone crash • Painful
Long-acting injection	Aveed 750 mg/mL	750 mg IM every 10 wk	• Long-acting • Consistent testosterone levels • Improved compliance	• Pain • Office injection • POMEs
Subcutaneous pellets	Testopel 75 mg/pellet	150–450 mg every 3–6 mo (manufacturer recommendation)	• Long-acting • Consistent testosterone levels • Improved compliance	• Office procedure • Expulsion • Infection • Pain

ORAL TESTOSTERONE PREPARATIONS

Orally administered testosterone is almost completely inactivated by first-pass metabolism by the liver metabolism. Oral 17-α-alkylated derivatives of testosterone decreases hepatic metabolism but can result in significant hepatotoxicity and lipid profile abnormalities. Newer testosterone agents have been developed to avoid hepatotoxicity, such as oral TU. TU must be taken with a fatty meal because it is absorbed into the lymphatic system and travels through the bloodstream and avoids the liver. The average dose is 120 to 240 mg/d and peaks in the circulation at 2 to 6 hours.[17] Oral TU is currently not available in the United States but is currently in phase 3 trials.

SUBCUTANEOUS TESTOSTERONE PELLETS

Subcutaneous pellets have been available for decades but were only FDA approved in 2008 (Testopel, Slate Pharmaceuticals). Testopel testosterone pellets are currently the only long-acting FDA approved pellet available in the United States. The pellets are placed under the skin in the fat layer through a simple office procedure. The pellets typically dissolve over 4 to 6 months. The pellets dissolve and thus do not need to be removed. Potential benefits of Testopel include that there is no risk for transference and improved patient compliance. There is also the convenience of not having a daily application. Potential risks of Testopel are bleeding, infection, expulsion of the pellets, pain, and bruising. In a multi-institutional study, Testopel provided sustained levels of testosterone for at least 4 months and up to 6 months in men with testosterone deficiency.[18] Implantation of more than 8 pellets achieved optimal results with respect to peak mean testosterone level and duration of effect. Testosterone pellets were generally well tolerated. Pharmacokinetic studies with Testopel have demonstrated that men with a body mass index (BMI) greater than 25 attained lower total testosterone peaks with slower decay than men with BMI less than 25. No differences were seen in decay rates for men with multiple implant rounds, and no differences in testosterone peaks or decay rates were seen in men with preimplantation testosterone level less than 300 or greater than or equal to 300 ng/dL.[19]

SHORT-ACTING TESTOSTERONE INJECTIONS

Currently available testosterone injection preparations include testosterone enanthate, cypionate, propionate, and undecanoate. Injectable testosterone first became available in the 1950s in the United States. IM administration of exogenous testosterone offers a cost-effective and efficacious method of TTh. The injectable testosterones have esterification of testosterone at the 17B-hydroxy position, which makes the compound more hydrophobic and allows for a longer duration of action. Peak serum concentrations are achieved within 72 hours, and injections are administered every 7 to 21 days, depending on symptom control, type of steroid, and androgen response in individual patients. Testosterone cypionate and testosterone enanthate are injected on average every 2 weeks and testosterone propionate 2 to 3 times per week due to its shorter half-life. The sudden decline of testosterone toward the end of the 2 to 3 weeks is also known as "testosterone crash," which is associated with a sudden and severe occurrence of hypogonadal symptoms. Patients taking injectable testosterone are more susceptible to erythrocytosis. One study found an increase in hematocrit (Hct) in 24% of patients after injections of testosterone cypionate without any adverse effects.[20] Older patients are much more likely to develop erythrocystosis, and caution should be taken in this population.

LONG-ACTING TESTOSTERONE INJECTIONS

Aveed is the only long-acting testosterone injection on the US market. Aveed contains 750 mg of TU, which is injected IM in 3 mL of castor oil.[14] TU is injected with a castor oil carrier, which enhances its ability to slow release over time.[21] Initial injection with Aveed requires a 4-week repeat injection. Following this initial repeat injection, Aveed is injected every 10 weeks. The most common adverse events associated with Aveed include acne and pain at the injection site. Rare cases of pulmonary oil microembolism (POME) have been reported, and thus, patients are required to remain in the doctor's office for 30 minutes to ensure POME does not occur.

TESTOSTERONE PATCHES

Patches were first introduced in 1994 as a scrotal patch (Testoderm) but were later discontinued due to scrotal irritation. Scrotal patches also associated with increased levels of DHT because the scrotum has high levels of 5 α-reductase. Later, nonscrotal testosterone patches (Androderm and Andropatch) were introduced. Androderm is available in a 2-mg and 4-mg patch. The patches are typically applied at night to the back, abdomen, thighs, or upper arms. The patches should be applied daily and at rotated sites to mitigate adverse skin reactions.

The patient should avoid showering, swimming, or washing the site for at least 3 hours after application.

Drawbacks of skin patches include their visibility and skin reaction. In fact, up to 30% of men can develop some type of skin reaction after applying these testosterone patches. Some studies have found that pretreating with 1% triamcinolone acetonide cream applied under the patch can decrease the risk of dermatitis without compromising testosterone absorption.[22] Some men have found benefit applying hydrocortisone cream on the affected area after removal of the patch. Other adverse reactions include skin induration, vesicle formation, allergic contact dermatitis, headaches, and depression.

ALTERNATIVES TO TESTOSTERONE THERAPY

Many young men with the diagnosis of hypogonadism desire testosterone therapy. However, exogenous testosterone acts like a natural contraceptive and thus should be avoided in these men. In these patients, it is recommended to use medications to increase their own endogenous testosterone and thus preserve, and possibly enhance, their fertility. The 3 most common mechanisms to raise endogenous testosterone are through the use of selective estrogen receptor modulators (SERMS), aromatase inhibitors (AIs), and human chorionic gonadotropin (hCG).

SERMs inhibit estrogen feedback to the hypothalamus, which in turn results in an increase in FSH and LH. SERMs also selectively modulate estrogen receptor subtypes and are unique in that they are not pure receptor agonists and antagonists but have variable effects depending on the tissue type. Clomiphene citrate is an SERM that is commonly used off-label in men to increase endogenous testosterone levels. Clomiphene is a SERM composed of a trans-isomer and longer acting zu-isomer, and it is typically administered as 25 mg or 50 mg daily or every other day. Studies have demonstrated that younger men are more responsive to clomiphene citrate than older men.[23] The most common side effects associated with clomiphene are hot flushes (10%), visual disturbances headaches, nausea, and vomiting.[24]

AIs inhibit the conversion from testosterone to estradiol and thus increase endogenous serum testosterone levels. Examples of AIs include letrozole, anastrozole, and testolactone. The main adverse event associated with AIs is the concern for bone health. There is controversy as to whether long-term use of AIs can adversely affect bone mineral density. Burnett-Bowie and colleagues[25] found that AIs led to a reduction in bone mineral density after 12 months, while others have found no change in bone resorption after 3 months of treatment.[26]

hCG is an LH analogue that stimulates Leydig cell production of testosterone. hCG is often administered IM or subcutaneously ranging from 500 IU every other day to 10,000 IU twice weekly. hCG has been shown to elevate testosterone levels into the normal therapeutic range. Tsujimura and colleagues[27] retrospectively analyzed 21 hypogonadal men using hCG injections. Low doses of hCG can stimulate and maintain spermatogenesis.[28] Adverse events associated with hCG include irritability, restlessness, edema, fatigue, headache, depression, injection site pain, and hypersensitivity reactions.[29]

EFFECTS OF LIFESTYLE INTERVENTIONS TO RAISE ENDOGENOUS TESTOSTERONE

Certain lifestyle changes can have a significant impact on raising endogenous testosterone levels. In a meta-analysis by Corona and colleagues,[30] they found that that both bariatric surgery and dietary interventions were associated with a significant increase in total and free testosterone. Increases in testosterone were greater in patients with bariatric surgery who also had greater weight loss. Another longitudinal study found that a greater than 15% loss in BMI was associated with a significant increase in total and free testosterone.[31] A study by Khoo and colleagues[32] found that moderate-intensity exercise also improves testosterone levels in a dose-dependent fashion in obese men. In this study, men treated with a mean 105 or 236 minutes of weekly exercise achieved time-dependent testosterone improvements (105 minutes = 22.8 ng/dL improvement; 236 minutes = 59.4 ng/dL improvement). Resistance exercise has also been shown to improve testosterone levels, with greater improvements noted in previously unconditioned men.[33–35]

ADVERSE EVENTS WITH TESTOSTERONE THERAPY

Serious adverse side effects secondary to testosterone administration are relatively uncommon if patients are monitored appropriately. Elderly patients seem to be more susceptible to experiencing adverse events with TTh. Many of the adverse events reported with TTh are primarily reported with supraphysiologic levels of testosterone. Often these adverse effects can be minimized by lowering the testosterone dosage, switching to an alternative form of therapy, or discontinuing TTh all together. Reported adverse effects include the following:

- Gynecomastia
- Erythrocytosis
- Prostate enlargement or exacerbation of BPH
- Hepatotoxicity (primarily with oral alkylated formulations)
- Impaired sperm production and fertility
- Edema
- Sleep apnea (primarily at supraphysiologic levels)
- Acne or oily skin

Erythrocytosis is the most common adverse event associated with TTh.[36] It seems that older men are at greatest risk for erythrocytosis. TTh can result in an increased risk of Hct greater than 50% (odds ratio 3.69, confidence interval 1.82–7.51), with a 3.2% mean increase noted over certain study intervals.[36,37] Guideline panels have recommended keeping Hct levels to less than 52% to 55% to prevent potential complications of hyperviscosity.[5,38]

Gynecomastia is a result of peripheral aromatization of testosterone to estradiol, which can increase breast tissue and cause breast pain. Patients with gynecomastia have benefited from either reducing the dose of testosterone or using estrogen receptor blockers such as tamoxifen.

FOLLOW-UP AND MONITORING

The goal of TTh is to alleviate hypogonadal symptoms by restoring physiologic levels of serum testosterone. However, the exact serum testosterone levels required to achieve optimal efficacy and safety is currently unknown.[39] Patients should be evaluated at 3 months after initiation of TTh and then every 6 to 12 months thereafter to assess serum testosterone levels, symptomatic improvement, PSA and digital rectal exam (DRE) changes, and changes in Hct. If an Hct level increases to greater than 54%, treatment options include discontinuation of TTh, therapeutic phlebotomy, or consideration of switching to another testosterone formulation if they are taking testosterone injections. Repeat bone dual-energy x-ray absorptiometry (DEXA) scan is indicated after 1 to 2 years of TTh in hypogonadal men with osteoporosis or low-trauma fractures. Patients failing to experience symptomatic improvement after 3 to 6 months of TTh despite adequate serum testosterone levels should discontinue TTh.

SUMMARY

Currently, there are numerous testosterone preparations available each with unique characteristics. Clinicians and patients should take into account cost, patient compliance, convenience, and ability to achieve appropriate serum testosterone concentrations when deciding which formulation to use. Other considerations before initiating TTh include the risk of transference and the desire to achieve a pregnancy in the future. TThs are constantly being developed for this growing market with future potential therapies, including newer SERMs, Oral testosterone undecanoate, stem cells, and nanotechnology.[40]

REFERENCES

1. Hoberman JM, Yesalis CE. The history of synthetic testosterone. Sci Am 1995;272(2):76–81.
2. Miller NL, Fulmer BR. Injection, ligation and transplantation: the search for the glandular fountain of youth. J Urol 2007;177(6):2000–5.
3. FDA. Drug safety communication. 2015. Available at: http://www.accessdata.fda.gov/scripts/cder/drugsatfda/index.cfm?fuseaction=Search.Search.
4. Grober ED, Khera M, Soni SD, et al. Efficacy of changing testosterone gel preparations (Androgel or Testim) among suboptimally responsive hypogonadal men. Int J Impot Res 2008;20(2):213–7.
5. Bhasin S, Cunningham GR, Hayes FJ, et al. Testosterone therapy in men with androgen deficiency syndromes: an Endocrine Society clinical practice guideline. J Clin Endocrinol Metab 2010;95(6):2536–59.
6. Basaria S, Dobs AS. New modalities of transdermal testosterone replacement. Treat Endocrinol 2003;2(1):1–9.
7. Swerdloff RS, Wang C, Cunningham G, et al. Long-term pharmacokinetics of transdermal testosterone gel in hypogonadal men. J Clin Endocrinol Metab 2000;85(12):4500–10.
8. Kaufman JM, Miller MG, Fitzpatrick S, et al. One-year efficacy and safety study of a 1.62% testosterone gel in hypogonadal men: results of a 182-day open-label extension of a 6-month double-blind study. J Sex Med 2012;9(4):1149–61.
9. Steidle C, Schwartz S, Jacoby K, et al. AA2500 testosterone gel normalizes androgen levels in aging males with improvements in body composition and sexual function. J Clin Endocrinol Metab 2003;88(6):2673–81.
10. Marbury T, Hamill E, Bachand R, et al. Evaluation of the pharmacokinetic profiles of the new testosterone topical gel formulation, Testim, compared to AndroGel. Biopharm Drug Dispos 2003;24(3):115–20.

11. Stahlman J, Britto M, Fitzpatrick S, et al. Effects of skin washing on systemic absorption of testosterone in hypogonadal males after administration of 1.62% testosterone gel. Curr Med Res Opin 2012;28(2): 271–9.

12. Dobs AS, McGettigan J, Norwood P, et al. A novel testosterone 2% gel for the treatment of hypogonadal males. J Androl 2012;33(4):601–7.

13. Upsher-Smith. Prescribing information. 2014. Available at: http://www.upsher-smith.com/wp-content/uploads/Vogelxo-MI.pdf.

14. Endo. Prescribing information. 2014. Available at: http://www.endo.com/File%20Library/Products/Prescribing%20Information/AVEED_prescribing_information.html.

15. Fabbri A, Giannetta E, Lenzi A, et al. Testosterone treatment to mimic hormone physiology in androgen replacement therapy. A view on testosterone gel and other preparations available. Expert Opin Biol Ther 2007;7(7):1093–106.

16. Kim S, Snipes W, Hodgen GD, et al. Pharmacokinetics of a single dose of buccal testosterone. Contraception 1995;52(5):313–6.

17. Gooren LJ. A ten-year safety study of the oral androgen testosterone undecanoate. J Androl 1994; 15(3):212–5.

18. McCullough AR, Khera M, Goldstein I, et al. A multi-institutional observational study of testosterone levels after testosterone pellet (Testopel(®)) insertion. J Sex Med 2012;9(2):594–601.

19. Pastuszak AW, Mittakanti H, Liu JS, et al. Pharmacokinetic evaluation and dosing of subcutaneous testosterone pellets. J Androl 2012;33(5): 927–37.

20. Sih R, Morley JE, Kaiser FE, et al. Testosterone replacement in older hypogonadal men: a 12-month randomized controlled trial. J Clin Endocrinol Metab 1997;82(6):1661–7.

21. Behre HM, Abshagen K, Oettel M, et al. Intramuscular injection of testosterone undecanoate for the treatment of male hypogonadism: phase I studies. Eur J Endocrinol 1999;140(5):414–9.

22. Cummings DE, Kumar N, Bardin CW, et al. Prostate-sparing effects in primates of the potent androgen 7alpha-methyl-19-nortestosterone: a potential alternative to testosterone for androgen replacement and male contraception. J Clin Endocrinol Metab 1998;83(12):4212–9.

23. Tenover JS, Bremner WJ. The effects of normal aging on the response of the pituitary-gonadal axis to chronic clomiphene administration in men. J Androl 1991;12(4):258–63.

24. Hill S, Arutchelvam V, Quinton R. Enclomiphene, an estrogen receptor antagonist for the treatment of testosterone deficiency in men. IDrugs 2009;12(2): 109–19.

25. Burnett-Bowie SA, McKay EA, Lee H, et al. Effects of aromatase inhibition on bone mineral density and bone turnover in older men with low testosterone levels. J Clin Endocrinol Metab 2009;94(12): 4785–92.

26. Leder BZ, Finkelstein JS. Effect of aromatase inhibition on bone metabolism in elderly hypogonadal men. Osteoporos Int 2005;16(12):1487–94.

27. Tsujimura A, Matsumiya K, Miyagawa Y, et al. Comparative study on evaluation methods for serum testosterone level for PADAM diagnosis. Int J Impot Res 2005;17(3):259–63.

28. Roth MY, Page ST, Lin K, et al. Dose-dependent increase in intratesticular testosterone by very low-dose human chorionic gonadotropin in normal men with experimental gonadotropin deficiency. J Clin Endocrinol Metab 2010;95(8):3806–13.

29. FDA. Human chorionic gonadotropin adverse effects. 2013. Available at: http://dailymed.nlm.nih.gov/dailymed/lookup.cfm. Accessed Nov 7, 2013.

30. Corona G, Rastrelli G, Monami M, et al. Body weight loss reverts obesity-associated hypogonadotropic hypogonadism: a systematic review and meta-analysis. Eur J Endocrinol 2013;168(6):829–43.

31. Camacho EM, Huhtaniemi IT, O'Neill TW, et al. Age-associated changes in hypothalamic-pituitary-testicular function in middle-aged and older men are modified by weight change and lifestyle factors: longitudinal results from the European male ageing study. Eur J Endocrinol 2013;168(3):445–55.

32. Khoo J, Tian HH, Tan B, et al. Comparing effects of low- and high-volume moderate-intensity exercise on sexual function and testosterone in obese men. J Sex Med 2013;10(7):1823–32.

33. Cadore EL, Lhullier FL, Alberton CL, et al. Salivary hormonal responses to different water-based exercise protocols in young and elderly men. J Strength Cond Res 2009;23(9):2695–701.

34. Cadore EL, Lhullier FL, Brentano MA, et al. Hormonal responses to resistance exercise in long-term trained and untrained middle-aged men. J Strength Cond Res 2008;22(5):1617–24.

35. Ahtiainen JP, Pakarinen A, Kraemer WJ, et al. Acute hormonal responses to heavy resistance exercise in strength athletes versus nonathletes. Can J Appl Physiol 2004;29(5):527–43.

36. Calof OM, Singh AB, Lee ML, et al. Adverse events associated with testosterone replacement in middle-aged and older men: a meta-analysis of randomized, placebo-controlled trials. J Gerontol A Biol Sci Med Sci 2005;60(11):1451–7.

37. Fernandez-Balsells MM, Murad MH, Lane M, et al. Clinical review 1: adverse effects of testosterone therapy in adult men: a systematic review and meta-analysis. J Clin Endocrinol Metab 2010;95(6): 2560–75.

38. Wang C, Nieschlag E, Swerdloff R, et al. Investigation, treatment and monitoring of late-onset hypogonadism in males: ISA, ISSAM, EAU, EAA and ASA recommendations. Eur J Endocrinol 2008;159(5): 507–14.

39. Wang C, Nieschlag E, Swerdloff RS, et al. ISA, ISSAM, EAU, EAA and ASA recommendations: investigation, treatment and monitoring of late-onset hypogonadism in males. Aging Male 2009; 12(1):5–12.

40. Ferrati S, Nicolov E, Zabre E, et al. The nanochannel delivery system for constant testosterone replacement therapy. J Sex Med 2015;12(6): 1375–80.

Testosterone and Male Infertility

Samuel J. Ohlander, MD, Mark C. Lindgren, MD, Larry I. Lipshultz, MD*

KEYWORDS

- Hypogonadism • Infertility • Hypogonadotropic • Testosterone • Exogenous • Spermatogenesis

KEY POINTS

- Multiple endogenous causes of hypogonadism may adversely affect a man's fertility potential.
- Fertility potential in the hypogonadal male may be reestablished through medical or surgical therapies, depending on the pathology.
- Exogenous testosterone is a known and common cause of infertility in men.
- Exogenous testosterone should be discontinued in any male trying to achieve pregnancy. Supplemental therapy to stimulate spermatogenesis may be necessary.

INTRODUCTION

Infertility is the inability to conceive after 12 months of unprotected intercourse. Approximately 15% of couples have infertility, but only 1 in 5 of these couples seek evaluation and treatment.[1] In 30% of infertile couples, a significant male factor alone is found as the cause for infertility. An additional 20% of couples have both male and female factors; therefore, male factors contribute to one-half of all infertile relationships. Endocrinopathies, including hypogonadism, are a common underlying problem in the infertile male, representing 9.6% of men presenting for infertility evaluation.[2] The many endogenous causes of hypogonadism are listed in **Box 1** and discussed in this paper. Exogenous testosterone, either prescribed by a physician or acquired by the patient elsewhere, is another commonly encountered cause of infertility. This paper discusses both exogenous testosterone and endogenous causes of hypogonadism as they relate to male infertility.

CAUSES OF HYPOGONADISM

Male patients presenting with infertility and no history of exogenous testosterone use may have an underlying endocrinopathy resulting in hypogonadism (low testosterone). The American Urological Association Best Practice Statement recommends testing serum testosterone and follicle-stimulating hormone (FSH) if the patient has oligozoospermia (especially if the sperm concentration is <10 million/mL), impaired sexual function, or if the patient has other clinical findings suggestive of an endocrinopathy.[3] Some physicians advocate a more extensive initial hormonal panel to include serum estradiol, luteinizing hormone (LH), sex hormone binding globulin, albumin, and/or prolactin.

The presence of testosterone is critical for spermatogenesis. Normal intratesticular testosterone levels are 50 to 100 times the concentration of testosterone found in serum.[4] The interference with this high level of intratesticular testosterone is one of the reasons exogenous testosterone can either greatly impair or shut down spermatogenesis entirely (**Fig. 1**). Likewise, endogenous hypogonadal states can be a cause for impaired spermatogenesis, and patients with hypogonadism can present with oligozoospermia or azoospermia.

Disclosure Statement: S.J. Ohlander and M.C. Lindgren have nothing to disclose. L.I. Lipshultz: Boston Scientific/American Medical Systems (Speaker, Consultant); Endo Pharmaceuticals (Consultant); Repros Medical (Clinical Investigator, Speaker, Consultant).
Division of Male Reproductive Medicine and Surgery, Scott Department of Urology, Baylor College of Medicine, Houston, TX 77030, USA
* Corresponding author. 6624 Fannin Street, Suite 1700, Houston, TX 77030.
E-mail address: larryl@bcm.edu

Urol Clin N Am 43 (2016) 195–202
http://dx.doi.org/10.1016/j.ucl.2016.01.006
0094-0143/16/$ – see front matter © 2016 Elsevier Inc. All rights reserved.

Hypogonadism is categorized as being either primary or secondary. Primary hypogonadism is failure at the level of the testis that is manifested by low serum testosterone and elevated gonadotropins (LH and FSH). Primary hypogonadism is also known as hypergonadotropic hypogonadism or primary testicular failure. Secondary hypogonadism, on the other hand, is hypogonadism in the setting of low or low normal gonadotropins, which is aptly named hypogonadotropic hypogonadism (HH).

Hypogonadotropic Hypogonadism

HH can be either congenital or owing to a variety of conditions that impair the hypothalamus or pituitary from properly releasing important trophic hormones for the testis. The hypothalamus releases gonadotropin-releasing hormone (GnRH) in pulsatile fashion to stimulate pituitary gonadotropes, which produce LH and FSH. Diseases or conditions that affect the pituitary and/or hypothalamus, including tumors, trauma, autoimmune disease, infarction, or infection, can disrupt gonadotropic function and lead to HH.[5]

Kallmann syndrome
The most common congenital form of HH results from the failure of GnRH-releasing neurons to

migrate to the olfactory lobe during development. An associated failure in development of the olfactory lobe leads to anosmia. Congenital anosmia and HH are the hallmarks of Kallmann syndrome, a cause of male infertility and, more rarely, female infertility, that occurs in 1 in 10,000 to 60,000 live births.[6] Patients commonly present after failing to undergo puberty, but may also have midline facial defects, congenital deafness, cranial asymmetry, cryptorchidism, or renal abnormalities.

Multiple genetic mutations have been implicated in cases of Kallmann syndrome, which lead to a variety of inheritance patterns. These gene mutations include those in the X-linked KAL1 gene and the autosomal-dominant fibroblast growth factor receptor 1 gene, known as FGFR1 or KAL2.[6,7] An additional gene coding for a G-protein–coupled receptor, PROKR2 or PROK2, have been found with apparent loss-of-function mutations leading to rare sporadic cases of Kallmann syndrome.[8] These known gene mutations have only been found in fewer than one-third of cases, which underscores the need for further study of this rare condition.[9]

Treatment of the delayed puberty and infertility associated with Kallmann syndrome is achieved by coordinated administration of gonadotropins. Testosterone therapy is used to initiate puberty in these patients, and, later, human chorionic gonadotropin (hCG) and human menopause gonadotropin (hMG) are used to induce spermatogenesis. With treatment, these patients can undergo adequate virilization and bone growth and many achieve pregnancy without the need for assisted reproductive technologies.[10]

Prader–Willi syndrome
Prader–Willi Syndrome affects approximately 1 in 15,000 to 1 in 30,000 individuals and is characterized by excessive appetite, obesity, mental

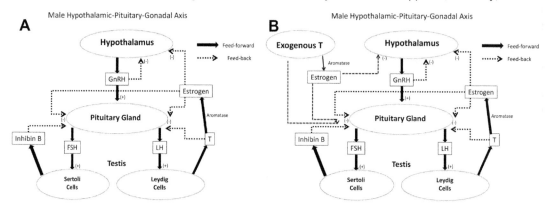

Fig. 1. Exogenous testosterone (T) causes increased negative feedback to the hypothalamus and pituitary, which decreases gonadotropins and endogenous production. (A, B) Male hypothalamic–pituitary–gonadal axis. GnRH, gonadotropin-releasing hormone; FSH, follicle-stimulating hormone; LH, luteinizing hormone.

retardation, cryptorchidism, infantile hypotonia, and HH.[11] It is most commonly caused by mutations or deletions of the paternally derived chromosome 15 at q11 or q13.[12,13] It is uncommon for these patients to seek infertility treatment.

Other genetic causes

A variety of genetic defects have been linked to HH. An X-linked gene, DAX1, is related to hypothalamic, pituitary, adrenal, and gonadal development, as well as maintaining spermatogenesis. DAX1 mutations can cause HH as well as congenital adrenal hyperplasia.[14] In patients with HH, numerous loss-of-function mutations have been identified in GnRHR, the gene that encodes the GnRH receptor found on pituitary gonadotropes.[15] Additionally, mutations have been found in the gene that encodes LH as well as the LH receptor, both of which have been found to cause hypogonadism in subfertile males.[16–18]

Hyperprolactinemia

The presence of excess serum prolactin inhibits LH action on Leydig cells, thereby causing hypogonadism. According to the American Urological Association Best Practice Statement, a serum prolactin measurement should be obtained if the patient's testosterone level is found to be low.[3] Hyperprolactinemia may be owing to a pituitary adenoma and warrants further workup. A careful history and physical examination should include questions about headaches, visual disturbances, galactorrhea, decreased libido, erectile dysfunction, as well as evaluation for visual field defects. MRI of the pituitary can further characterize the lesion as either a macroadenoma, 1 cm or larger in its greatest dimension, or a microadenoma, less than 1 cm or normal imaging. Approximately one-third of men with hyperprolactinemia are found to have macroadenomas of the pituitary, which are more likely to lead to mass effect symptoms, such as headaches or visual field defects.[19]

Treatment of hyperprolactinemia depends on the size of the lesion. Microadenomas are treated with dopamine agonists, which suppress the production of prolactin. Cabergoline has become the standard of care for such lesions with superior efficacy and a more acceptable side effect profile when compared with bromocriptine.[19] Traditionally, the presence of a macroadenoma was indication for surgical resection. Advances in surgical and endoscopic approaches to resection have led to decreased invasiveness and potential morbidity from this surgery. Despite this, some macroadenomas are initially treated medically with surgical excision reserved for patients who fail treatment.[20] With treatment, patients have been shown to have normalized testosterone levels, improved libido, and better erectile function, as well as improvements in sperm count.[21]

Congenital Adrenal Hyperplasia

Congenital adrenal hyperplasia is caused by a variety of enzyme defects in the steroidogenesis pathway, with 21-hydroxylase deficiency accounting for the majority of cases.[22] The resultant downstream deficiency of cortisol production causes the pituitary to release excessive adrenocorticotropic hormone, which further stimulates the adrenal gland, leading to hyperplasia. As a result of the deficient steroidogenic pathway, an excess of adrenal androgens is produced. These androgenic hormones suppress pituitary release of gonadotropins, which leads to decreased testicular production of testosterone and impaired fertility. The phenotype of men with congenital adrenal hyperplasia is very variable and depends on the degree of androgen excess. Some congenital adrenal hyperplasia patients with a mild phenotype are capable of achieving pregnancy with no treatment, whereas others require treatment to maximize their fertility potential.[22]

Hyperestrogenemia

Estrogen is an important negative feedback signal in the hypothalamic–pituitary–gonadal (HPG) axis. Testosterone, produced by the testis, is converted to estradiol by aromatase in peripheral tissues. Estradiol then acts directly on the hypothalamus and pituitary, via the estrogen receptor, giving a strong inhibitory signal that suppresses the release of GnRH, FSH, and LH. In addition to the HPG axis suppression, estrogen in excess can directly impair spermatogenesis.[23] Men with hyperestrogenemia are found to have low serum FSH, LH, and testosterone in the setting of elevated serum estradiol.

Hyperestrogenemia may be owing to liver failure or tumors that produce estrogen, but it is most commonly caused by obesity. Increased adipose tissue, which contains aromatase, leads to increased conversion of testosterone to estradiol. Aromatase inhibitors can both decrease the hyperestrogenemia and increase testosterone levels. Additionally, weight loss has been shown to improve the testosterone/estrogen balance.[24–27]

Klinefelter Syndrome

Patients with Klinefelter syndrome have an extra X chromosome (47,XXY) owing to a nondisjunction event that usually happens during meiosis of either the paternal or maternal gamete. These patients often present to the infertility specialist with nonobstructive azoospermia. In fact, up to 10% of patients presenting with nonobstructive azoospermia have Klinefelter syndrome, which makes it the most common genetic cause for nonobstructive azoospermia.[28] The original description by Klinefelter in 1942 included hypergonadotropic hypogonadism, gynecomastia, and infertility.[29] Additionally, the phenotype can include tall stature, decreased virilization, mild cognitive impairment, and small testes. Up to 10% of Klinefelter patients have a mosaic pattern with cells containing either 46,XY or 47,XXY, owing to a mitotic nondisjunction during embryogenesis.[30] For patients with this mosaic pattern, it is possible to have sperm in the ejaculate, albeit typically at severely oligozoospermic levels.

The mechanism by which Klinefelter patients are azoospermic or oligozoospermic is multifactorial, with hypogonadism probably playing a part. Regardless, microsurgical testicular sperm extraction has become the standard of care for Klinefelter patients with sperm retrieval rates ranging as high as 69%.[31–33] Sperm extraction techniques coupled with in vitro fertilization and intracytoplasmic sperm injection have had high fertilization rates in Klinefelter patients. However, patients must be counseled that the XXY genotype and Klinefelter syndrome may be passed to the offspring.[34,35] Additionally, preimplantation genetic diagnosis techniques should be considered to limit the risk of Klinefelter syndrome in the offspring.

HYPOGONADISM AND EXOGENOUS TESTOSTERONE

Male patients presenting with both infertility and exogenous testosterone use have become increasingly common. The number of men seeking infertility treatment after having been treated for symptomatic hypogonadism has skyrocketed in recent years, in part because of the variety of new testosterone formulations that are now available and the associated marketing efforts of the pharmaceutical industry that have resulted in a more than 170% increase in sales over the last 5 years.[36] Unfortunately, not all hypogonadal men are receiving appropriate consultation on the fertility implications of treatment. In addition to patients treated for hypogonadism, infertile men may also present with a history of anabolic–androgenic steroid (AAS) use. As many as 20% of legally sold sports nutrition supplements in the United States contain synthetic AAS.[37,38] The average, naïve consumer may not realize that these over-the-counter supplements can have a negative impact on their fertility potential.

The next section discusses the impact exogenous testosterone can have on fertility, the management of infertile men taking testosterone, and strategies to maintain or recover spermatogenesis in patients who are to be treated with testosterone.

PRESERVATION OF SPERMATOGENESIS

Before the initiation of hormonal therapy, the potential negative impact on a man's fertility must be discussed, particularly when that therapy includes exogenous testosterone. Before initiating testosterone therapy in a young patient, it is our practice to thoroughly discuss the risks and benefits and obtain written consent, as well as obtain a baseline semen analysis.

With an increased awareness for men's health, hypogonadism is being diagnosed more commonly outside of the setting of an infertility workup. Recent publications have demonstrated the negative impact of hypogonadism on cardiovascular mortality, metabolic syndrome, non–insulin-dependent diabetes, and depression, thus supporting the benefits of therapy.[39–41] Additionally, a 2014 metaanalysis by Sagoe and colleagues[42] identified a 6.4% global lifetime prevalence of AAS use among males. Coward and colleagues[43] found that almost one-half of men presenting for treatment of profound hypogonadism (<50 ng/dL) identified prior AAS use as the etiology. Unfortunately, 15% of men presenting with AAS-induced hypogonadism reported regret of their use of steroids, and a significant number cited a lack of understanding of the fertility implications as their reason for regret.[44]

Exogenous testosterone, a known male contraceptive, has been prescribed by well-meaning, but woefully misinformed physicians as a treatment for infertility in hypogonadal men. A survey among American Urologic Association members found that 25% of urologists prescribed testosterone for the treatment of infertility in the hypogonadal male, suggesting a misunderstanding of the HPG axis.[45] For men taking exogenous testosterone, spontaneous recovery of spermatogenesis has been noted to occur 4 to 12 months after cessation, but recovery is not guaranteed.[46] In a study by Anderson and Wu,[47] 70% of men developed azoospermia or severe oligozoospermia after 18 months of exogenous testosterone therapy with only 85% experiencing fertility potential upon cessation. The World Health Organization similarly found that with cessation of injectable testosterone after 6 months of use, only 46% of men achieved their baseline semen parameters.[48] Complex fertility and hormone management requires the evaluation and care of a specialist.

Once the decision is made to treat the symptomatic hypogonadal male, the patient and physician must have a thorough discussion about family planning. Certain scenarios exist: the male whose family is complete, or does not wish to preserve future fertility; the male who wishes to preserve future fertility, but is not actively trying to reproduce; the male who is actively trying to achieve a pregnancy; and the male who has been on testosterone therapy and is looking to recover spermatogenesis. For the male who does not wish to preserve his fertility, treatment will not require maintenance of spermatogenesis. This section focuses on men who wish to preserve or recover fertility potential.

We strongly recommend a semen analysis before the initiation of hormonal therapy to establish baseline semen parameters. For the male who wishes to pursue a family more than 1 year from the time of initiating therapy, we recommend concurrent hormonal therapy with testosterone replacement and hCG. As an analog of LH, hCG stimulates the secretion of testosterone from Leydig cells. Depenbusch and colleagues[49] initially demonstrated the ability of hCG to maintain spermatogenesis in a study of 13 men with idiopathic hypogonadism, Kallmann syndrome, or pituitary insufficiency in which spermatogenesis was induced with either GnRH or hCG/hMG. The patients were then administered additional hCG for the maintenance of secondary sexual characteristics. After 12 months of therapy, 12 of the 13 patients had preserved spermatogenesis, although with diminished sperm counts. Later, Hsieh and colleagues[50] demonstrated preservation of spermatogenesis with low-dose hCG (500 IU intramuscular every other day) in men on topical or injectable testosterone therapy. Semen parameters were followed in 2- to 4-month intervals with no significant changes from pretreatment parameters after 360 days of follow-up. Subset analysis did not demonstrate a difference between topical and intramuscular applications. Upon the couple's decision to pursue a pregnancy, the therapy regimen must then be modified to optimize spermatogenesis, which requires cessation of exogenous testosterone.

RECOVERY OF SPERMATOGENESIS

The initial step in the recovery of spermatogenesis should be the discontinuation of exogenous testosterone. As previously noted, cessation alone does not always result in recovery of semen parameters that meet the World Health Organization criteria. Additionally, stopping testosterone therapy may result in return of the symptoms that

required treatment. Abrupt cessation without means of hormonal supplementation often results in severe hypogonadism until the body has recovered its baseline physiologic production.

Early studies by Vicari and colleagues[51] demonstrated recovery of spermatogenesis in 13 of 17 previously azoospermic patients using hCG alone. Subsequent administration of hMG in the same cohort demonstrated limited further improvement in semen parameters. Of the 10 patients attempting to conceive, 2 of the 4 patients produced a pregnancy with hCG alone, and 5 of 6 men with hCG/hMG produced a pregnancy despite limited objective evidence of improved fertility potential.

Recently, Wenker and colleagues[52] published a report of 49 men with azoospermia or severe oligozoospermia (<1 million/mL) secondary to testosterone therapy (mean time of therapy of 52 months) who were placed on hCG combination therapy. Testosterone therapy was discontinued and the patients were placed on a regimen of hCG with supplemental medications to support FSH production. To sustain stable levels, hCG was dosed at 3000 IU subcutaneously every other day. Coadministration of clomiphene citrate (71.4% of patients), tamoxifen (57.1%), anastrozole (20.4%), or recombinant FSH (2%) to support endogenous production of FSH was provided for a mean duration of 14 months. Of the 49 subjects, 47 demonstrated a return of spermatogenesis or improvement over the 1 million/mL density, and more than one-third of patients achieved a pregnancy. The mean time to return of spermatogenesis was approximately 4 months for injection and transdermal applications of testosterone. Upon the return of spermatogenesis for these patients, the first semen analysis had a mean sperm density of 22.6 million/mL. For patients who have been on extended testosterone therapy, our practice is to initiate 3000 IU of hCG subcutaneously every other day with 25 mg of clomiphene citrate daily to recover spermatogenesis upon the cessation of testosterone therapy.

Should adequate recovery of spermatogenesis not occur after 6 months of therapy, we include subcutaneous injection of recombinant FSH at 75 to 150 IU 3 times per week. An initial case report by Kliesch and colleagues[53] demonstrated recovery of sperm in the ejaculate after 18 weeks of combination therapy of hCG and recombinant FSH in a male with azoospermia secondary to pituitary insufficiency owing to surgical management of prolactinoma. Additional studies have supported the findings of Kliesch and colleagues,[54,55] demonstrating induction of spermatogenesis in azoospermic, hypogonadal men following failure of therapy with HCG alone. Further work by

Matsumoto and colleagues[56] demonstrated recovery of spermatogenesis in 29 azoospermic males with HH with combination hCG and recombinant FSH. After 18 weeks of therapy, 80% of patients established a sperm density of 1.5×10^6/mL and 27% of men established concentrations of greater than 20×10^6/mL. Five of the 29 patients achieved a clinical pregnancy.

SUMMARY

Hypogonadism and its therapies have a significant impact on male fertility potential. It is necessary to determine the etiology to treat and counsel the patient appropriately regarding therapeutic options. For the hypogonadal male on exogenous testosterone, management should begin with cessation of the exogenous testosterone therapy and initiation of treatment with supplemental subcutaneous hCG and an oral FSH-inducing agent to allow reestablishment of the HPG axis and spermatogenesis. Further supplemental therapy with recombinant FSH may be necessary to achieve optimal semen parameters in some patients.

REFERENCES

1. Sharlip ID, Jarow JP, Belker AM, et al. Best practice policies for male infertility. Fertil Steril 2002;77(5): 873–82.
2. Sigman M, Jarow JP. Endocrine evaluation of infertile men. Urology 1997;50(5):659–64.
3. Practice Committee of American Society for Reproductive Medicine. Diagnostic evaluation of the infertile male: a committee opinion. Fertil Steril 2012; 98(2):294–301.
4. Coviello AD, Matsumoto AM, Bremner WJ, et al. Low-dose human chorionic gonadotropin maintains intratesticular testosterone in normal men with testosterone-induced gonadotropin suppression. J Clin Endocrinol Metab 2005;90(5):2595–602.
5. Seminara SB, Oliveira LM, Beranova M, et al. Genetics of hypogonadotropic hypogonadism. J Endocrinol Invest 2000;23(9):560–5.
6. Tsai PS, Gill JC. Mechanisms of disease: insights into X-linked and autosomal-dominant Kallmann syndrome. Nat Clin Pract Endocrinol Metab 2006; 2(3):160–71.
7. Hershkovitz E, Loewenthal N, Peretz A, et al. Testicular expressed genes are missing in familial X-Linked Kallmann syndrome due to two large different deletions in daughter's X chromosomes. Horm Res 2008;69(5):276–83.
8. Leroy C, Fouveaut C, Leclercq S, et al. Biallelic mutations in the prokineticin-2 gene in two sporadic cases of Kallmann syndrome. Eur J Hum Genet 2008;16(7):865–8.
9. Dode C, Hardelin JP. Kallmann syndrome. Eur J Hum Genet 2009;17(2):139–46.
10. Sigman M. Assisted reproductive technics for the treatment of male factor infertility. R I Med J 1991; 74(12):591–6.
11. Cassidy SB, Driscoll DJ. Prader-Willi syndrome. Eur J Hum Genet 2009;17(1):3–13.
12. Burman P, Ritzen EM, Lindgren AC. Endocrine dysfunction in Prader-Willi syndrome: a review with special reference to GH. Endocr Rev 2001;22(6): 787–99.
13. Smeets DF, Hamel BC, Nelen MR, et al. Prader-Willi syndrome and Angelman syndrome in cousins from a family with a translocation between chromosomes 6 and 15. N Engl J Med 1992;326(12):807–11.
14. Burris TP, Guo W, McCabe ER. The gene responsible for adrenal hypoplasia congenita, DAX-1, encodes a nuclear hormone receptor that defines a new class within the superfamily. Recent Prog Horm Res 1996;51:241–59 [discussion: 259–60].
15. Bedecarrats GY, Kaiser UB. Mutations in the human gonadotropin-releasing hormone receptor: insights into receptor biology and function. Semin Reprod Med 2007;25(5):368–78.
16. Huhtaniemi I. The Parkes lecture. Mutations of gonadotrophin and gonadotrophin receptor genes: what do they teach us about reproductive physiology? J Reprod Fertil 2000;119(2):173–86.
17. Wu RH, Rosenfeld R, Fukushima D. Hypogonadism and Leydig cell hypoplasia unresponsive to human luteinizing hormone (hLH). Am J Med Sci 1984; 287(3):23–5.
18. Wu SM, Hallermeier KM, Laue L, et al. Inactivation of the luteinizing hormone/chorionic gonadotropin receptor by an insertional mutation in Leydig cell hypoplasia. Mol Endocrinol 1998;12(11):1651–60.
19. Gillam MP, Molitch ME, Lombardi G, et al. Advances in the treatment of prolactinomas. Endocr Rev 2006; 27(5):485–534.
20. Shimon I, Benbassat C, Hadani M. Effectiveness of long-term cabergoline treatment for giant prolactinoma: study of 12 men. Eur J Endocrinol 2007; 156(2):225–31.
21. De Rosa M, Ciccarelli A, Zarrilli S, et al. The treatment with cabergoline for 24 month normalizes the quality of seminal fluid in hyperprolactinaemic males. Clin Endocrinol (Oxf) 2006;64(3):307–13.
22. Urban MD, Lee PA, Migeon CJ. Adult height and fertility in men with congenital virilizing adrenal hyperplasia. N Engl J Med 1978;299(25):1392–6.
23. Hammoud Z, Tan B, Badve S, et al. Estrogen promotes tumor progression in a genetically defined mouse model of lung adenocarcinoma. Endocr Relat Cancer 2008;15(2):475–83.
24. Giagulli VA, Kaufman JM, Vermeulen A. Pathogenesis of the decreased androgen levels in obese men. J Clin Endocrinol Metab 1994;79(4):997–1000.

25. Globerman H, Shen-Orr Z, Karnieli E, et al. Inhibin B in men with severe obesity and after weight reduction following gastroplasty. Endocr Res 2005;31(1): 17–26.

26. Kaukua J, Pekkarinen T, Sane T, et al. Sex hormones and sexual function in obese men losing weight. Obes Res 2003;11(6):689–94.

27. Tchernof A, Despres JP, Belanger A, et al. Reduced testosterone and adrenal C19 steroid levels in obese men. Metabolism 1995;44(4):513–9.

28. Oates RD. Clinical and diagnostic features of patients with suspected Klinefelter syndrome. J Androl 2003; 24(1):49–50.

29. Klinefelter HF. Syndrome characterized by gynecomastia, aspermatogenesis without a-leydigism, and increased excretion of follicle-stimulating hormone. J Clin Endocrinol Metab 1942;2(11):615–24.

30. Therman E. Human chromosomes: structure, behavior, and effects. New York: Springer-Verlag; 1993.

31. Madgar I, Dor J, Weissenberg R, et al. Prognostic value of the clinical and laboratory evaluation in patients with nonmosaic Klinefelter syndrome who are receiving assisted reproductive therapy. Fertil Steril 2002;77(6):1167–9.

32. Schiff JD, Palermo GD, Veeck LL, et al. Success of testicular sperm extraction [corrected] and intracytoplasmic sperm injection in men with Klinefelter syndrome. J Clin Endocrinol Metab 2005;90(11): 6263–7.

33. Westlander G, Ekerhovd E, Granberg S, et al. Testicular ultrasonography and extended chromosome analysis in men with nonmosaic Klinefelter syndrome: a prospective study of possible predictive factors for successful sperm recovery. Fertil Steril 2001;75(6):1102–5.

34. Komori S, Horiuchi I, Hamada Y, et al. Birth of healthy neonates after intracytoplasmic injection of ejaculated or testicular spermatozoa from men with nonmosaic Klinefelter's syndrome: a report of 2 cases. J Reprod Med 2004;49(2):126–30.

35. Ron-El R, Raziel A, Strassburger D, et al. Birth of healthy male twins after intracytoplasmic sperm injection of frozen-thawed testicular spermatozoa from a patient with nonmosaic Klinefelter syndrome. Fertil Steril 2000;74(4):832–3.

36. Layton JB, Li D, Meier CR, et al. Testosterone lab testing and initiation in the United Kingdom and the United States, 2000 to 2011. J Clin Endocrinol Metab 2014;99(3):835–42.

37. Baume N, Mahler N, Kamber M, et al. Research of stimulants and anabolic steroids in dietary supplements. Scand J Med Sci Sports 2006;16(1):41–8.

38. Geyer H, Parr MK, Koehler K, et al. Nutritional supplements cross-contaminated and faked with doping substances. J Mass Spectrom 2008;43(7): 892–902.

39. Corona G, Monami M, Rastrelli G, et al. Testosterone and metabolic syndrome: a meta-analysis study. J Sex Med 2011;8(1):272–83.

40. Corona G, Rastrelli G, Monami M, et al. Hypogonadism as a risk factor for cardiovascular mortality in men: a meta-analytic study. Eur J Endocrinol 2011; 165(5):687–701.

41. Zarrouf FA, Artz S, Griffith J, et al. Testosterone and depression: systematic review and meta-analysis. J Psychiatr Pract 2009;15(4):289–305.

42. Sagoe D, Molde H, Andreassen CS, et al. The global epidemiology of anabolic-androgenic steroid use: a meta-analysis and meta-regression analysis. Ann Epidemiol 2014;24(5):383–98.

43. Coward RM, Rajanahally S, Kovac JR, et al. Anabolic steroid induced hypogonadism in young men. J Urol 2013;190(6):2200–5.

44. Kovac JR, Scovell J, Ramasamy R, et al. Men regret anabolic steroid use due to a lack of comprehension regarding the consequences on future fertility. Andrologia 2015;47(8):872–8.

45. Samplaski MK, Loai Y, Wong K, et al. Testosterone use in the male infertility population: prescribing patterns and effects on semen and hormonal parameters. Fertil Steril 2014;101(1):64–9.

46. Turek PJ, Williams RH, Gilbaugh JH 3rd, et al. The reversibility of anabolic steroid-induced azoospermia. J Urol 1995;153(5):1628–30.

47. Anderson RA, Wu FC. Comparison between testosterone enanthate-induced azoospermia and oligozoospermia in a male contraceptive study. II. Pharmacokinetics and pharmacodynamics of once weekly administration of testosterone enanthate. J Clin Endocrinol Metab 1996;81(3): 896–901.

48. Contraceptive efficacy of testosterone-induced azoospermia in normal men. World Health Organization Task Force on methods for the regulation of male fertility. Lancet 1990;336(8721): 955–9.

49. Depenbusch M, von Eckardstein S, Simoni M, et al. Maintenance of spermatogenesis in hypogonadotropic hypogonadal men with human chorionic gonadotropin alone. Eur J Endocrinol 2002;147(5): 617–24.

50. Hsieh TC, Pastuszak AW, Hwang K, et al. Concomitant intramuscular human chorionic gonadotropin preserves spermatogenesis in men undergoing testosterone replacement therapy. J Urol 2013; 189(2):647–50.

51. Vicari E, Mongioi A, Calogero AE, et al. Therapy with human chorionic gonadotrophin alone induces spermatogenesis in men with isolated hypogonadotrophic hypogonadism–long-term follow-up. Int J Androl 1992;15(4):320–9.

52. Wenker EP, Dupree JM, Langille GM, et al. The use of HCG-based combination therapy for recovery of

spermatogenesis after testosterone use. J Sex Med 2015;12(6):1334–7.

53. Kliesch S, Behre HM, Nieschlag E. Recombinant human follicle-stimulating hormone and human chorionic gonadotropin for induction of spermatogenesis in a hypogonadotropic male. Fertil Steril 1995; 63(6):1326–8.

54. Bouloux PM, Nieschlag E, Burger HG, et al. Induction of spermatogenesis by recombinant follicle-stimulating hormone (puregon) in hypogonadotropic azoospermic men who failed to respond to human chorionic gonadotropin alone. J Androl 2003;24(4):604–11.

55. Liu PY, Turner L, Rushford D, et al. Efficacy and safety of recombinant human follicle stimulating hormone (Gonal-F) with urinary human chorionic gonadotrophin for induction of spermatogenesis and fertility in gonadotrophin-deficient men. Hum Reprod 1999;14(6):1540–5.

56. Matsumoto AM, Snyder PJ, Bhasin S, et al. Stimulation of spermatogenesis with recombinant human follicle-stimulating hormone (follitropin alfa; GONAL-f): long-term treatment in azoospermic men with hypogonadotropic hypogonadism. Fertil Steril 2009;92(3):979–90.

Testosterone Deficiency and the Prostate

Joseph P. Alukal, MD*, Herbert Lepor, MD

KEYWORDS

- Testosterone deficiency • Benign prostatic hyperplasia • Prostate cancer • Dihydrotestosterone
- Sexual development

KEY POINTS

- Testosterone and dihydrotestosterone are important to normal prostate development and function.
- Blockade of dihydrotestosterone production results in reduced prostate size and reduced risk of prostate cancer.
- Testosterone supplementation may alter prostate size.
- Further study of the prostate and its relationship to testosterone physiology is warranted.

INTRODUCTION

The prostate is a male reproductive organ of both endodermal and mesodermal origin; it is located in the pelvis, immediately superior to the muscles of the pelvic floor. The prostate is intimately associated with the bladder neck and the posterior urethra, which it encircles. It has both a glandular and muscular component, which enables it to perform its unique function with respect to ejaculation. Prostatic secretions from the glandular component comprise most of the seminal fluid that is ejaculated; coordinated contractions of the muscular component (along with the muscles of the pelvic floor and the bladder neck) enable antegrade ejaculation of seminal fluid. The observation that the prostate is centrally important to reproductive function is an accurate one.

The growth and development of the functioning prostate depends on the actions of testosterone and its metabolite dihydrotestosterone (DHT). These two potent hormones enable in particular the growth and proliferation of the glandular component of the prostate through binding and activation of androgen receptor (AR) within the cytoplasm of prostatic epithelial cells.[1] Extensive research has established that the activation of this receptor also enables proliferative growth of this component, which in turn causes benign prostatic hyperplasia (BPH); in addition, this pathway enables carcinogenesis within prostatic epithelial cells, leading to prostate cancer (PCa).[2–4] Both diseases are common and burdensome conditions in aging men.[5,6] However, the relationship between testosterone and these two conditions is unclear; hypogonadism (low testosterone level), BPH, and PCa are all age-related conditions.

This article reviews the existing data regarding these relationships. Pharmacologic treatments for both conditions depend on manipulation of these pathways; this article reviews these treatments, as well as outlining future directions for treatment that are being explored. In addition, the need for further research into the nature of these two conditions is reviewed.

EMBRYOLOGY OF THE PROSTATE

Prostate development is an early fetal event in all male mammals; in humans this event occurs at 10 to 12 weeks.[7] The prostate arises from the urogenital sinus, which consists of an epithelial

Department of Urology, New York University School of Medicine, 150 East 32nd Street, Second Floor, New York, NY 10016, USA
* Corresponding author.
E-mail address: Joseph.alukal@nyumc.org

Urol Clin N Am 43 (2016) 203–208
http://dx.doi.org/10.1016/j.ucl.2016.01.013

layer (derived from endoderm) surrounded by a mesenchymal layer derived from mesoderm. Invagination of the epithelial folds into the mesenchyme results in the glandular architecture of the prostate.[8] The proliferation of these epithelial cells occurs under the influence of testosterone.[7]

Levels of testosterone in the male fetus are high; postpartum, this increase in testosterone level persists into the second year of life. Testosterone is also constantly being converted by the intracellular enzyme 5-alpha reductase (5-AR) into DHT.[7] DHT is a more potent activator of AR, binding to the receptor with a 10-fold greater affinity.[9] In the male fetus, DHT drives organogenesis of both the male external genitalia and the prostate. As testosterone levels decrease after the second year of life, DHT levels decrease correspondingly. High levels of 5-AR are found within cells of the prostatic epithelium as well as follicular cells of the scalp. This second fact is important given the observation the DHT levels in part drive male pattern baldness.[10]

Disruptions in these pathways can result in abnormal sexual differentiation and ambiguous genitalia; these intersex conditions are characterized by predictable phenotypes that relate to the disruption in question. For example, testicular feminization syndrome is characterized by normal-appearing female external genitalia.[11] This condition is caused on a cellular level by absent or nonfunctioning AR. In spite of increased testosterone and DHT levels, the cellular changes that result from activated AR do not occur. Importantly, patients with testicular feminization syndrome fail to develop a prostate (because of the absence of DHT activity). They do develop a normal female external phenotype because of conversion of testosterone into estrogen through action of the enzyme aromatase. This process, aromatization, is the only source of estrogen in male patients, and represents an important pathway for metabolism of testosterone. Aromatase is found in lipid cells, and aromatization can therefore be a more robust effect in obese patients. Patients with testicular feminization have a rudimentary vagina; however, there is an absent uterus, cervix, and proximal vagina. These structures fail to develop under the influence of a müllerian inhibiting substance (MIS), another important regulator of reproductive organogenesis in the fetus.[12] MIS is normally produced in the Sertoli cells of the male testis; in patients with testicular feminization, the testis is present (albeit undescended) and partly functional. The local actions of MIS in both types of patient (and the normal male fetus) include driving the regression of müllerian duct structures (which normally develop into the proximal portion of the vagina, the cervix, the uterus, and the fallopian tubes).[13]

Another condition that shows the role of AR in reproductive development is 5-alpha reductase deficiency, an autosomal recessive disease recognized in a small population of men from the Dominican Republic.[14] 5-AR–deficient patients are born phenotypically female, again in spite of normal levels of testosterone. The absence of activity of 5-AR results in deficient levels of DHT; without DHT there is a failure to drive organogenesis of normal male external genitalia. Normal production of MIS by Sertoli cells of the testis again results in regression of müllerian duct structures. During puberty, the larger spike in testosterone levels drives the development of a male external phenotype through adequate activation of AR (even without measurable levels of DHT). The result is that these patients are born appearing female, but eventually develop a male appearance. This phenomenon is recognized within this community and the transition these children make during puberty is anticipated as being fairly common. The absence of DHT throughout the adult life of these patients results in other important phenotypic traits. These patients are highly unlikely to develop urinary symptoms because of BPH, and they are less likely to develop prostate cancer or male pattern baldness.[15]

Other conditions resulting in incomplete virilization are well described, most importantly congenital adrenal hyperplasia.[16] In this spectrum of conditions resulting in varying degrees of ambiguous genitalia, there are defects in the steroid biosynthesis of testosterone. The result is varying deficiencies in terms of testosterone production as well as DHT levels (See Patricia Freitas Corradi, Renato B. Corradi, Loren Wissner Greene: Physiology of the Hypothalamic Pituitary Gonadal Axis in the Male, in this issue for further details).

TESTOSTERONE AND PROSTATE GROWTH (PUBERTY, MIDDLE AGE, OLD AGE)

As boys enter puberty just after the age of 10 years, testosterone and DHT levels spike again in a predictable fashion, assuming an intact hypothalamic-pituitary-gonadal axis. This event drives the physical changes associated with sexual maturity as well as the onset of reproductive maturity[17]; spermatogonial stem cells in the testis begin to undergo meiotic division into spermatozoa. In the prostate, proliferation of prostatic epithelial cells initiates a period of prostate growth; in addition, prostatic secretion from these cells begins and patients begin to experience seminal emission.[18]

These processes are again driven by the influence of testosterone and DHT; much of what is understood about this process was observed in 5-AR–deficient patients who undergo a transition from phenotypic femaleness to maleness during puberty. In these patients, the massive spike in testosterone level that occurs with puberty does not correspond with a spike in DHT level, because there is no conversion of testosterone to DHT occurring through 5-AR. Activation of the AR with increased levels of testosterone alone is enough to drive the transition to phenotypic maleness and progression through puberty; increase in prostate size and size of external genitalia, development of pubic and axillary hair, as well as growth of muscle and bone all occur to near-normal degrees in 5-AR–deficient men.[14] However, the fundamental difference in prostate physiology in these patients is one of slower growth and decreased risk of prostate cancer throughout later life. It was this observation that drove researchers to investigate 5-AR blockade as a pharmacologic mechanism for treatment of BPH as well as prostate cancer prevention.[15]

TESTOSTERONE AND BENIGN PROSTATIC HYPERPLASIA

BPH is a common problem affecting all men as they age.[19] The Urologic Disease in America project, published in 2005, characterized the public health burden of BPH; in the year 2000, across all urology providers in the United States, there were 4.5 million physician visits related to a primary diagnosis of BPH and 368 ambulatory surgery procedures performed for every 100,000 visits.[20] The relationship between BPH and associated lower urinary tract symptoms (LUTS) is not exactly linear; although patients are more likely to develop LUTS as their prostates enlarge, this is not guaranteed.[21] In addition, some patients with LUTS caused by prostatic obstruction have small prostates. Regardless, pharmacologic mechanisms for decreasing prostate size have long represented a high-yield target for the management of LUTS in male patients.

The first commercially available 5-AR inhibitor was finasteride (Proscar, Propecia, Merck); at a 5-mg daily dose, this drug represents a first-line treatment of LUTS caused by BPH. The drug was released in 1992; the Medical Therapy of Prostatic Symptoms (MTOPS) trial, published in 2003, clearly showed that finasteride treatment resulted in a significant decrease in prostate size. In addition, finasteride, when added to monotherapy for BPH/LUTS with an α-blocker, resulted in symptom improvement.[21] Long-term follow-up studies confirmed the initial effect observed in this trial in terms of prostate size decrease.[22]

Since this time, a second 5-AR inhibitor was released, dutasteride (Avodart, GSK). This drug has some theoretic increase in efficacy attributable to its binding of all 3 isoforms of 5-AR within prostate epithelial cells, whereas finasteride binds only 2 of 3 isoforms of 5-AR.[23] No clinical head-to-head studies were performed.

Both drugs capitalize on the relationship between DHT and prostate growth first identified in 5-AR–deficient patients; blockade of 5-AR in prostate epithelial cells results in prevention of DHT production. This prevention in turn removes a key driver of prostate growth. Testosterone levels in these patients remain unchanged (there is a small increase observed in testosterone levels) and prostate size shrinks regardless, which confirms that DHT is the key driver in BPH.

Numerous studies over the years have confirmed the relationship between testosterone replacement and BPH[24,25]; the various formulations of testosterone that are currently commercially available all include warnings regarding worsening of urinary symptoms on initiation of therapy. However, in all likelihood, the driving force behind this relationship is conversion of the increased/supplemented testosterone into DHT, with the corresponding increase in DHT level driving BPH and worsening urinary symptoms in some, but not all, patients.

TESTOSTERONE AND PROSTATE CANCER

The data regarding the relationship between testosterone and prostate cancer are numerous and varied in terms of their implications (See Emily Davidson, Abraham Morgentaler: Testosterone Therapy and Prostate Cancer, in this issue). However, one aspect of this complex relationship is well shown by the studies examining 5-AR inhibitors.

Two large, prospective, randomized, placebo controlled trials were performed examining the relationship between chronic 5-AR inhibitor usage and prostate cancer incidence: The Reduction by Dutasteride of Prostate Cancer Events (REDUCE) trial and the Prostate Cancer Prevention Trial (PCPT).[26,27] Both studies showed an approximate 30% risk reduction in the development of prostate cancer over the 10-year period of the study. Some initial concern regarding slight increases in high-risk cancers in the treatment arms of both studies was dismissed initially as being most likely caused by detection bias (as opposed to treatment effect); the long-term follow-up of the PCPT, published in 2013, supported this theory, at least in so far as disease-specific mortality in the treatment arm was far less than in the placebo arm (implying no meaningful increase in high-risk, clinically significant cancers with 5-AR inhibitor use).[28]

The conclusion reached is therefore that (1) DHT levels can in part drive prostate carcinogenesis; and that (2) decreasing these levels, in addition to preventing prostate enlargement, can prevent prostate cancer. The corresponding question of whether testosterone levels themselves influence prostate cancer risk remains unanswered. Numerous data exist regarding this specific question; they point to different conclusions. Some studies implicate low testosterone levels as conferring a higher likelihood of high-risk prostate cancer, implying that more than 1 pathway for prostate carcinogenesis might exist.[29,30] The data regarding management of metastatic prostate cancer through chemical castration further support the relationship between testosterone levels and prostate cancer progression.[31] Further discussion of that relationship, which is also complex, follows elsewhere in this issue (See Emily Davidson, Abraham Morgentaler: Testosterone Therapy and Prostate Cancer, in this issue).

Regardless, given that low testosterone levels should correlate with low DHT levels, it is reasonable to think that the observations from the trials discussed earlier would hold and that hypogonadal patients would be less likely to develop any kind of prostate cancer. Instead, the common epidemiologic observation that both prostate cancer and low testosterone levels are diseases of aging men confounds this picture.[19] A man in his 80s is far more likely to have both low testosterone level and prostate cancer than he was in his 20s. Whether or not this observation is correlative but not causal remains to be proved. Given the common and burdensome nature of both problems, further study is warranted.

FUTURE DIRECTIONS

Numerous avenues for further investigation into this topic remain open. First, many of the large studies evaluating prostate size and treatment with either testosterone or 5-AR inhibitors depend on transrectal ultrasonography for measurement of prostate volume. This modality is highly variable; inexact measurements can be obtained for several reasons, including operator variability and patient discomfort. Second, prostate cancer incidence in both the REDUCE and PCPT trials was determined using transrectal ultrasonography–guided prostate needle biopsy. This modality is also inexact. Data at our institution and elsewhere

establish clearly that both prostate volume measurement and prostate cancer detection are improved with use of multiparametric MRI of the prostate.[32] Follow-up studies incorporating MRI as a means of following prostate volume change and development of prostate cancer might help illuminate the true effect of testosterone and DHT within the prostate.

Assays of testosterone and DHT represent a source of variability as well; both measurements are subject to diurnal variability (testosterone levels to a greater degree) and this introduces a further source of inaccuracy to the existing data. "Who is the truly hypogonadal patient?" is a question that first needs to be answered before figuring out whether or not the patient is at increased or reduced risk of prostate cancer. Assays of AR function at the cellular level, including the upregulation of downstream genetic targets of activated AR, could represent a future means to more accurately distinguish hypogonadal from eugonadal patients.

In addition, data from another study published in 2015 by Finkelstein and colleagues[33] showed that the understanding of hypogonadism as a disease driven only by testosterone levels is incomplete. Patients enrolled in this study were eugonadal; they were initially treated with a gonadotropin-releasing hormone receptor agonist (leuprolide), which subsequently resulted in castrate levels of testosterone. They were then given varying degrees of testosterone replacement; some were replaced to therapeutic levels, some to subtherapeutic or supratherapeutic levels. They were also randomized to treatment with an aromatase inhibitor (anastrozole) or a placebo; blockade of aromatization in the treatment arm resulted in absent levels of estrogen in these patients, and this was in spite of normal or near-normal testosterone levels. Unexpectedly, some patients in the treatment arm, again with normal testosterone levels and low estrogen levels, complained of symptoms that are normally attributed to low testosterone levels (central obesity, fatigue, low libido). This effect could only be explained by the inadequate levels of estrogen in these patients. Previously, no data existed that implicated estrogen levels in men in any of these processes.

The idea that testosterone, DHT, and estrogen are all powerful hormones with effects on male physiology is incompletely understood at best. The relationship between these 3 hormones within the prostate and the possibility that different patients respond differently to these hormones at the cellular level (in much the same way that estrogen and progesterone have different cellular effects in some women with regard to breast cancer) warrants further investigation.

SUMMARY

The relationship between testosterone and prostate health is centrally important to men's health. Prostate growth, sexual and reproductive function, the risk of prostate cancer, and the likelihood of urinary symptoms related to prostate obstruction; all of these men's health issues are in some fashion related to testosterone. Although the existing data are extensive and illuminate this many-faceted relationship, understanding of the pathways by which testosterone and the prostate influence each other is incomplete. Further research is warranted given the central importance of prostate health to the male population.

REFERENCES

1. Anderson KM, Liao S. Selective retention of dihydrotestosterone by prostatic nuclei. Nature 1968; 219(5151):277–9.
2. Chodak GW, Kranc DM, Puy LA, et al. Nuclear localization of androgen receptor in heterogeneous samples of normal, hyperplastic and neoplastic human prostate. J Urol 1992;147(3 Pt 2):798–803.
3. Lesser B, Bruchovsky N. The effects of testosterone, 5α-dihydrotestosterone and adenosine 3',5'-monophosphate on cell proliferation and differentiation in rat prostate. Biochim Biophys Acta 1973; 308(3):426–37.
4. Huggins C, Hodges CV. Studies on prostatic cancer. Cancer Res 1941;1:297.
5. Wei JT, Calhoun E, Jacobsen SJ. Urologic diseases in America project: benign prostatic hyperplasia. J Urol 2005;173(4):1256–61.
6. Available at: http://www.cdc.gov/cancer/prostate/statistics.
7. Randall VA. 9 Role of 5α-reductase in health and disease. Baillieres Clin Endocrinol Metab 1994;8(2): 405–31.
8. Aumüller G. Morphologic and endocrine aspects of prostatic function. Prostate 1983;4(2):195–214.
9. Grino PB, Griffin JE, Wilson JD. Testosterone at high concentrations interacts with the human androgen receptor similarly to dihydrotestosterone. Endocrinology 1990;126(2):1165–72. DHT AR activity (MTOPS list?).
10. Kaufman KD, Olsen EA, Whiting D, et al. Finasteride in the treatment of men with androgenetic alopecia. J Am Acad Dermatol 1998;39(4):578–89.
11. Morris JM. The syndrome of testicular feminization in male pseudohermaphrodites. Am J Obstet Gynecol 1953;65(6):1192–211.
12. Teixeira J, Maheswaran S, Donahoe PK. Mullerian inhibiting substance: an instructive developmental hormone with diagnostic and possible therapeutic applications. Endocr Rev 2001;22(5):657–74.
13. Donahoe PK, Ito Y, Hendren WH. A graded organ culture assay for the detection of Mullerian inhibiting substance. J Surg Res 1977;23(2):141–8.
14. Imperato-McGinley J, Guerrero L, Gautier T, et al. Steroid 5α-reductase deficiency in man: an inherited form of male pseudohermaphroditism. Science 1974;186(4170):1213–5.
15. Bautista OM, Kusek JW, Nyberg LM, et al. Study design of the Medical Therapy of Prostatic Symptoms (MTOPS) trial. Control Clin trials 2003;24(2): 224–43.
16. White PC, New MI, Dupont BO. Congenital adrenal hyperplasia. N Engl J Med 1987;316(25):1580–6.
17. August GP, Grumbach MM, Kaplan SL. Hormonal changes in puberty: III. correlation of plasma testosterone, LH, FSH, testicular size, and bone age with male pubertal development. J Clin Endocrinol Metab 1972;34(2):319–26.
18. Isaacs JT. Antagonistic effect of androgen on prostatic cell death. Prostate 1984;5(5):545–57.
19. Kupelian V, Wei JT, O'Leary MP, et al. Prevalence of lower urinary tract symptoms and effect on quality of life in a racially and ethnically diverse random sample: the Boston Area Community Health (BACH) Survey. Arch Intern Med 2006; 166(21):2381–7.
20. Litwin MS, Saigal CS, Yano EM, et al. Urologic Diseases in America Project: analytical methods and principal findings. J Urol 2005;173(3):933–7.
21. McConnell JD, Roehrborn CG, Bautista OM, Medical Therapy of Prostatic Symptoms (MTOPS) Research Group. The long-term effect of doxazosin, finasteride, and combination therapy on the clinical progression of benign prostatic hyperplasia. N Engl J Med 2003; 349(25):2387–98.
22. Roehrborn CG. BPH progression: concept and key learning from MTOPS, ALTESS, COMBAT, and ALF-ONE. BJU Int 2008;101(s3):17–21.
23. Roehrborn CG, Boyle P, Nickel JC, et al. Efficacy and safety of a dual inhibitor of 5-alpha-reductase types 1 and 2 (dutasteride) in men with benign prostatic hyperplasia. Urology 2002;60(3):434–41.
24. Tenover JS. Effects of testosterone supplementation in the aging male. J Clin Endocrinol Metab 1992; 75(4):1092–8.
25. Behre HM, Bohmeyer J, Nieschlag E. Prostate volume in testosterone-treated and untreated hypogonadal men in comparison to age-matched normal controls. Clin Endocrinol 1994; 40(3):341–9.
26. Andriole G, Bostwick D, Brawley O, et al, REDUCE Study Group. Chemoprevention of prostate cancer in men at high risk: rationale and design of the Reduction by Dutasteride of Prostate Cancer Events (REDUCE) trial. J Urol 2004; 172(4):1314–7.

27. Thompson IM, Goodman PJ, Tangen CM, et al. The influence of finasteride on the development of prostate cancer. N Engl J Med 2003;349(3):215–24.

28. Thompson IM Jr, Goodman PJ, Tangen CM, et al. Long-term survival of participants in the prostate cancer prevention trial. N Engl J Med 2013;369(7): 603–10.

29. Morgentaler A, Rhoden EL. Prevalence of prostate cancer among hypogonadal men with prostate-specific antigen levels of 4.0 ng/mL or less. Urology 2006;68(6):1263–7.

30. Mearini L, Zucchi A, Nunzi E, et al. Low serum testosterone levels are predictive of prostate cancer. World J Urol 2013;31(2):247–52.

31. Crawford ED, Eisenberger MA, McLeod DG, et al. A controlled trial of leuprolide with and without fluta-mide in prostatic carcinoma. N Engl J Med 1989; 321(7):419–24.

32. Wysock JS, Rosenkrantz AB, Huang WC, et al. A prospective, blinded comparison of magnetic resonance (MR) imaging–ultrasound fusion and vi-sual estimation in the performance of MR-targeted prostate biopsy: the PROFUS trial. Eur Urol 2014; 66(2):343–51.

33. Finkelstein JS, Lee H, Burnett-Bowie SAM, et al. Gonadal steroids and body composition, strength, and sexual function in men. N Engl J Med 2013; 369(11):1011–22.

Testosterone Therapy and Prostate Cancer

Emily Davidson, BS, Abraham Morgentaler, MD*

KEYWORDS

- Testosterone • Prostate • Prostate cancer • Androgens • Prostate-specific antigen
- Testosterone deficiency • Hypogonadism

KEY POINTS

- Considerable evidence contradicts the notion that higher testosterone levels are associated with increased risk of developing prostate cancer, or higher grade Gleason score.
- Major changes in prostate-specific antigens are observed when a serum testosterone moves into or out of the castrate range, but are not observed for changes at higher concentrations.
- Testosterone therapy may now be considered for selected men with a history of prostate cancer, provided that informed consent is obtained and close monitoring is performed.

INTRODUCTION

The biological effects of testosterone have been recognized throughout the recorded history of humankind, even before identification of the key biochemical element produced by the testis. With so much debate surrounding the use of testosterone therapy and prostate cancer, the entire background must be clear. The scientific history of testosterone started in 1849 with Arnold Berthold. Through his experiments with rooster castration and subsequent testes transplantation, he linked the physiologic and behavioral changes of castration to a substance secreted by the testes.[1] More interest developed as Dr Charles E. Brown-Séquard made a presentation on the self-administration of *liquid testiculaire* at the Societé de Biologie in June of 1889. He reported that the injection of testicular extracts derived from dogs and guinea pigs resulted in his increased physical strength, mental abilities, and appetite.[2] Scientists around the world continued to experiment with testicular extracts and testicular "transplants" as treatment for the maladies of aging. Finally, testosterone was isolated by David and colleagues[3] in 1935 and synthesized later that year. Both Adolf Butenandt and Leopold Ruzicka were awarded with the Nobel Prize for Chemistry in 1939 for their work.

Initially, there was an early 'honeymoon period' for testosterone therapy after it first became available, shortly after its synthesis.[4] An article from 1940 in the *New England Journal of Medicine* noted improvements in sexual desire and performance, increased strength, and improved sense of well-being in men treated for hypogonadism.[5] This 'honeymoon period' was short lived, as Huggins and Hodges reported in 1941 that castration caused regression of metastatic prostate cancer, and testosterone injections "activated" prostate cancer,[6] based on alterations in the prostate cancer serum marker, acid phosphatase. From that point on, use of testosterone became rare owing to fear of causing prostate cancer in otherwise healthy individuals.

Disclosure Statement: Dr A. Morgentaler has received payments for research, consulting, lecture honoraria, and/or scientific advisory boards for AbbVie, Antares, Bayer, Clarus, Eli Lilly (27705), Endo (201107293), and Pfizer. Ms E. Davidson has no conflicts to declare.
Men's Health Boston, Department of Surgery (Urology), Harvard Medical School, 200 Boylston Street, Suite A309, Chestnut Hill, MA 02467, USA
* Corresponding author.
E-mail address: dr.morgentaler@menshealthboston.com

Urol Clin N Am 43 (2016) 209–216
http://dx.doi.org/10.1016/j.ucl.2016.01.007
0094-0143/16/$ – see front matter © 2016 Elsevier Inc. All rights reserved.

The Modern Era of Testosterone Therapy

Before the early 1990s, the use of testosterone therapy was rare, and was limited almost exclusively to younger men with severe cases of testosterone deficiency (TD) owing to pituitary tumors, anorchia, or genetic abnormalities such as Klinefelter syndrome. Over the past 20 years there has been a remarkable and steady growth in the use of testosterone therapy. This has occurred as a result of increased physician awareness of TD and the benefits of treatment, together with increased convenience of testosterone formulations.[7] Notable benefits include improved sexual desire and performance, improved energy, increased muscle and bone density, and improved metabolic status, similar to benefits reported at the advent of testosterone use in the 1940s.[5,8] The reinvigorated interest in testosterone therapy has led to a reexamination of traditional assumptions concerning prostate cancer and testosterone.[9] Despite important advances in our understanding of this topic, the use of testosterone therapy continues to be controversial because of prostate cancer fears, and this remains the greatest concern among physicians around the world with regard to the use of testosterone therapy.[10]

The Androgen Hypothesis

Stemming from reports in the 1940s, the androgen hypothesis has come to include the following features: prostate cancer is an androgen-dependent cancer, high testosterone levels contribute to the development of prostate cancer, high testosterone causes rapid growth of prostate cancer, and low testosterone is protective against development of prostate cancer and causes prostate cancer to regress.[1,11–13] Ever since, medical students and physicians have been taught that high testosterone promotes prostate cancer development and there seemed to be no reason to doubt this axiomatic concept.[14] The relationship between testosterone and prostate cancer was classified as "fuel for a fire" or "food for a hungry tumor".[15] In an international survey published in 2007, as many as 70% of health care providers were concerned about the association of testosterone therapy and prostate cancer.[16] It was not until recently that this conventional wisdom was challenged.

The breakdown of the androgen hypothesis evolved throughout the years, beginning in the early 1990s. Morgentaler and colleagues[17] published a study in which testosterone deficient men with normal prostate-specific antigen (PSA; <4.0 ng/mL) and a normal digital rectal examination underwent a sextant prostate biopsy before initiating testosterone therapy. Interestingly, 11 of the first 77 men had prostate cancer. Compared with the 15.2% prostate cancer rate noted by Thompson and colleagues[18] in the placebo arm of the Prostate Cancer Prevention Trial, this 14.3% rate was shockingly similar. This was the first indication that low testosterone may be a risk factor for prostate cancer, and not protective against prostate cancer and its progression.[14]

Since this revelation, more than 20 population-based longitudinal studies have shown no relationship between prostate cancer and serum testosterone or other androgens.[19] The Endogenous Hormones and Prostate Cancer Collaborative Group published high-level evidence from a metaanalysis consisting of 18 studies that included 3886 men with incident prostate cancer and 6438 controls.[20] The results demonstrated no direct association between endogenous serum androgens and the development of prostate cancer. Additionally, Muller and colleagues[21] analyzed 3255 men in the placebo arm of the reduction by Dutasteride of Prostate Cancer Events trial. Men underwent prostate biopsies at 2 years and 4 years and there was no relationship found between testosterone or dihydrotestosterone levels and prostate cancer risk.

Although high testosterone levels were thought to contribute to the development of prostate cancer, there is a complete lack of compelling evidence in the literature.[22] An extensive review found that men with higher endogenous testosterone or who had undergone testosterone therapy were not at increased risk of prostate cancer.[20] Supraphysiologic doses of testosterone for up to 9 months in healthy men failed to demonstrate a significant increase in PSA or prostate volume.[23,24] The notion that "more testosterone is bad, less testosterone is good" was not necessarily true.

The Saturation Model

However, physicians still recognize that initiation of androgen deprivation causes rapid declines in PSA and that cessation of androgen deprivation causes rapid increases in PSA. Revisiting the landmark work of Huggins and Hodges, the traditional view suggests a continuous relationship between serum testosterone and prostate cancer growth.[15] Studies from Prout and Brewer[25] and Fowler and Whitmore[12] present an alternative possibility. Both papers noted no evidence of progression in men with prostate cancer not treated by androgen deprivation or castration.[12,25] The evidence presents a paradox: how can prostate cancer be so sensitive to androgen deprivation, yet seem to be indifferent to variations in serum androgens under other circumstances?

The resolution of this paradox is the saturation model. The saturation model accounts for the key observation that prostate tissue is exquisitely sensitive to changes in serum testosterone at low concentrations, but becomes indifferent to these changes at higher concentrations.[26] Exposure to increasing concentrations of androgen causes prostate tissue growth, but this growth rate plateaus when the concentration reaches a limit.[27] There exists a threshold (saturation point) beyond which there is no further ability to induce androgen-driven changes in prostate tissue growth.[9] Similar relationships are found throughout biology. This explains why dramatic PSA changes are noted when serum testosterone is manipulated into or out of the castration range, but minimal PSA changes occur when supraphysiologic testosterone doses are administered to normal men.[28]

At least 2 mechanisms underlie the model. The first is the finite ability of the androgen receptor to bind androgen.[29,30] Maximal binding of the androgen to the androgen receptor (saturation) in human prostate is achieved in vitro at approximately 4 nmol-1.[28] In vivo, the saturation point is approximately double this value, at 8nmol/L or approximately 250 ng/dl.[9] Because the primary actions of androgen on prostate tissue occur via binding to androgen receptor, once the androgen receptors are saturated the presence of higher androgen concentrations should not elicit further biochemical response.[26] A second mechanism is that intraprostatic androgen concentrations seem to be somewhat independent of serum concentrations.[28] Marks and colleagues[31] demonstrated that intraprostatic concentrations of testosterone and dihydrotestosterone were unchanged after 6 months of testosterone injections, despite large increases in serum testosterone concentrations. This raises the possibility that the prostate maintains a relatively homeostatic microenvironment with regards to androgens, relatively unaffected by changes in serum androgens.[26]

This saturation model derails the notion that testosterone is "fuel for a fire" or "food for a hungry tumor."[14] An analogy that better fits the available evidence is "testosterone is like water for a thirsty tumor." Once that thirst has been quenched by adequate testosterone concentrations, additional androgens serve as nothing more than excess.[27]

The presentation of the saturation model and the shift in concepts regarding testosterone and prostate cancer have important clinical implications. Approximately 20% to 30% of elderly men over the age of 60 experience TD.[32] Symptoms of TD vary, but include fatigue, weakness, decreased libido and energy, erectile dysfunction, reduced muscle and bone mass, and increased abdominal fat.[33] Testosterone therapy is an effective, commonly used treatment shown to be effective in mitigating the bothersome symptoms of TD.[34]

As physicians gain a better understanding of TD and its consequences, there has been a reevaluation of the risks of testosterone therapy, particularly with regard to prostate cancer. Some clinicians still fear that testosterone therapy may unmask occult prostate cancer in otherwise healthy men with TD, but more evidence is mounting in favor of the benefits of testosterone therapy.[34] Whereas prior history of prostate cancer was considered an absolute contraindication to the use of testosterone therapy, physicians are recognizing the benefits of testosterone treatment in certain populations.[33]

Although no randomized, controlled trials have been performed to assess testosterone therapy and prostate cancer risk, evidence to date fails to suggest increased risk.[9] Calof and colleagues[35] conducted a metaanalysis of 19 placebo-controlled testosterone therapy trials and found no significant increase in prostate cancer or development of PSA levels greater than 4.0 ng/ml in men treated with testosterone therapy versus placebo. A systematic review of 11 placebo-controlled studies by Shabsigh and colleagues[36] showed that men who received testosterone therapy had neither increased risk of prostate cancer nor greater Gleason grade among those who developed prostate cancer. In the UK Androgen study, Feneley and Carruthers[37] followed 1365 British men 28 to 87 years of age and found the risk of prostate cancer diagnosis to be similar to age-matched controls. Only 1 of 20 patients with high-grade prostatic intraepithelial neoplasia developed prostate cancer during 12 months of testosterone therapy.[38] Combined with the studies cited previously reporting no increased risk of prostate cancer based on endogenous androgen concentrations, these data can reliably ease the fear that higher testosterone concentrations increase the risk of prostate cancer.

Association of Low Serum Testosterone with Prostate Cancer

Clouded by the long-held fear that high serum testosterone is a risk for prostate cancer, there has been little appreciation for a literature that strongly shows a relationship between low serum testosterone concentrations and high-risk prostate cancer.[15] Men with the lowest tertile of serum testosterone had nearly double the risk of being diagnosed with prostate cancer on biopsy compared with men with less severe TD, in a study of 345 men with TD and PSA levels of less than 4.0 ng/mL.[18] Among men with prostate cancer, a high Gleason score has been reported with lower serum testosterone concentrations.[39,40] In an open clinical study conducted by Mearini and colleagues,[41] 37% of the 65 patients with prostate cancer had testosterone levels of less than 2.5 ng/mL. One study from García-Cruz and colleagues[42] including 137 men undergoing biopsy for suspicion of prostate cancer found an inverse relationship between serum testosterone and prostate cancer. Salonia and colleagues[43] measured serum testosterone on the day before radical prostatectomy (RP), and found that the risk of seminal vesicle invasion, a markedly poor prognostic indicator, was increased significantly in men with low testosterone levels, including a 3-fold increased risk in men with severely reduced serum testosterone.[14]

Low levels of serum testosterone have also been reported in association with poor prognosis from prostate cancer. Yamamoto and colleagues[44] reported increased rates of biochemical recurrence after RP in patients with low testosterone, and low levels of free testosterone were reported as an independent prognostic factor for prostate cancer progression in a study of 154 men undergoing active surveillance for prostate cancer.[45]

These studies are consistent with the epidemiology of prostate cancer, in that there is increased prevalence of high-grade prostate cancer as men age (Thompson and colleagues[18]) and testosterone levels decline.

Testosterone Therapy in Men with a History of Prostate Cancer

Testosterone therapy for men with a history of prostate cancer remains controversial, particularly because prostate cancer has been considered a contraindication for testosterone therapy for several decades, and testosterone product labels carry this warning as well. However, with the emergence of the saturation model and evidence mounting against the traditional androgen hypothesis, the paradigm has shifted. Multiple investigators have now reported on the use of testosterone therapy in men with prostate cancer, with published case series beginning in the mid-2000s. Overall, these studies have provided reassuring results regarding the risk of testosterone therapy in men with prostate cancer. In a study by Kaplan and Hu,[46] Surveillance, Epidemiology, and End Results data were linked to Medicare data to identify 149,354 men diagnosed with prostate cancer between 1992 and 2007. Of these, 1181 (0.79%) received testosterone therapy after diagnosis.

No differences were reported in overall survival, cancer-specific survival, or in the use of salvage androgen deprivation therapy in men with or without use of testosterone after diagnosis.

In 2004, Kaufman and Graydon[47] reported no prostate cancer recurrences in 7 men treated with testosterone therapy after RP. Median follow-up in the study was 2 years, with the longest follow-up of 12 years. Agarwal and Oefelein[48] reported no recurrences in 10 testosterone deficient men with history of RP who received testosterone therapy for up to 19 months. In a larger case series of 57 men with predominantly low and intermediate risk prostate cancer, Khera and colleagues[49] reported no biochemical recurrences after a median follow-up time of 13 months. Men were treated with testosterone therapy for an average of 36 months after RP. In the largest series to date, Pastuszak and colleagues[50] examined the records of 103 hypogonadal men after RP. In this study there were also 49 eugonadal men who underwent RP but did not receive testosterone therapy, included as a comparison group. Approximately one-quarter of these men in each group were considered high risk based on Gleason score 8 to 10, positive margins, or the presence of positive lymph nodes at surgery. With a median follow-up of 27 months, biochemical recurrence rates were 4% in the testosterone-treated group and 16% in the untreated, eugonadal group.

In 2007, Sarosdy[51] published a case series evaluating 31 men with TD receiving testosterone therapy after brachytherapy treatment for prostate cancer. The median time for initiation of testosterone therapy was 2 years after treatment and median follow-up was 5 years (range, 1.5–9). There was no evidence of biochemical recurrence and none of the men halted testosterone therapy owing to prostate cancer recurrence. Morales and colleagues[52] reported a prospective case series consisting of 5 men that had been previously treated with external beam radiation therapy for prostate cancer. After reaching nadir PSA levels, these men received testosterone therapy. Median follow-up was 14.5 months (range, 6–27). The PSA level did increase transiently in 1 patient, but none exceeded 1.5 ng/mL to raise any concern of biochemical recurrence.

A small number of reports also describe testosterone therapy in men who underwent radiation therapy for prostate cancer. In 2013, Pastuszak and colleagues[53] evaluated 13 men with low and intermediate risk prostate cancer treated with testosterone therapy after radiation (brachytherapy or external beam radiation therapy). After median follow-up of 29.7 months, no biochemical recurrences were reported. More recently,

Balbontin and colleagues[54] reported no biochemical recurrence in a case series of 20 men with low-risk prostate cancer treated with brachytherapy. Testosterone treatment lasted for a median of 14 months and median follow-up was 31 months (range, 12–48). Notably, PSA level declined from 0.7 to 0.1 ng/mL. More recently, Pastuszak and colleagues[55] also present a multiinstitutional cohort of 98 men who received testosterone therapy after radiation treatment for prostate cancer. Of these men, 76.6% had low or intermediate risk prostate cancer and the median follow-up was 40.8 months. A small but statistically significant increase in PSA levels was noted with testosterone therapy, from 0.8 to 0.9 mg/mL, and 6 men (6.1%) experienced biochemical recurrence. This recurrence rate is lower than previously reported rates of biochemical recurrence after radiation therapy. However, one must be cautious in drawing conclusions owing to the limited sample size of this and other studies, their retrospective study design, and single-arm methodology.

In addition, there are now several reports of testosterone therapy in men undergoing active surveillance for prostate cancer. Morgentaler and colleagues[56] performed a retrospective study of 13 hypogonadal men receiving testosterone therapy for at least 12 months while undergoing active surveillance for prostate cancer. Median follow-up was 2.5 years (range, 1–8.1). At initial biopsy, 12 men had low-risk prostate cancer and 1 man had intermediate risk prostate cancer (Gleason 3 + 4). No prostate cancer progression was noted, and no cancer was found in 54% of biopsies. Recently, Kacker and colleagues[57] retrospectively reviewed a larger series of men on active surveillance, comparing progression rates in 28 men with TD who underwent testosterone therapy with 96 men with TD who did not receive testosterone therapy. Median follow-up was 38.9 months and 42.4 months for the testosterone group and the no-testosterone groups, respectively. Progression rates were similar between the 2 groups.

A cautionary note was struck by Morales,[58] who reported erratic PSA responses to testosterone therapy in 6 men with untreated prostate cancer and one man without documented prostate cancer. However, no follow-up biopsy results were reported, making it difficult to interpret these results.[58]

Discussion

Given the proven benefits of testosterone therapy for testosterone-deficient men, clinicians are faced with a dilemma. Large numbers of men around the world, including younger men aged 40 to 50 years, have been treated and cured of prostate cancer. With some of these men having long life expectancies, is it reasonable to deprive these men of a treatment that may provide important benefits and enhanced quality of life based on a historical concern that does not seem to be supported by current scientific evidence?

When evidence contradicts theory, it is useful to try to understand how the theory came into being. From the early 1940s when Huggins first reported that castration lowered serum acid phosphatase in men and that testosterone injections increased it, there was extremely limited clinical experience with testosterone therapy. This situation changed with introduction of the first branded topical testosterone products in the late 1990s and early 2000s. Before that time, the only experience physicians had with manipulation of testosterone levels, particularly urologists, was to lower serum testosterone into the castrate range as treatment for prostate cancer. This effectively lowered PSA. There was no reason, therefore, to question the axiom that high testosterone contributed to prostate cancer development and growth, and that low testosterone protected against it. It was therefore stunning to discover in 2006 that the original conclusion by Huggins—that testosterone injections "activated" prostate cancer—was based on only a single hormonally intact patient. The reliable, albeit temporary, results observed by all urologists with lowering androgen concentrations, and the lack of experience with raising testosterone contributed to the belief that higher testosterone concentrations were risky.

Today, it must be recognized that there exists no evidence that testosterone therapy increases prostate cancer risk in testosterone-deficient men. Although the fear of aggravating prostate cancer with testosterone therapy among physicians is understandable given our training, it should be clear that the theoretic underpinning of this concept has been shown to be unsound, and there are now numerous clinical experiences and publications that demonstrate that the risk of worsening prostate cancer outcomes with testosterone therapy seems to be small, if present at all.

The leading controversy today is whether testosterone therapy can be safely offered to men with a history of prostate cancer. Recommendations for this have been provided in a recent review by a group of experts in the field.[9] Our own recommendations are similar. Candidates should be those with symptomatic TD who stand to benefit from treatment. Informed consent should be provided to patients, specifically including information that safety data are limited, no controlled prospective studies have yet been performed, and there is thus an unknown degree of risk of cancer progression or recurrence with testosterone therapy. We require a signed consent form stating these points in our practice. In addition, patients should be informed of the standard risks associated with testosterone therapy, including acne, erythrocytosis, fluid retention, peripheral edema, infertility, testicular atrophy, and gynecomastia.

It is useful to remember that prostate cancer recurrence occurs at a significant rate in men treated for prostate cancer, even if no testosterone therapy is offered. This baseline risk of approximately 15% must be considered when offering testosterone therapy. This means that some men will experience prostate cancer recurrence or progression whether or not they receive testosterone therapy. However, there will be a reflex presumption on the part of patients and other physicians that it was the increase in serum androgens that triggered the recurrence or progression. Adequate counseling of patients before beginning testosterone therapy is of great help in countering this eventuality, and we repeat this conversation regularly during the course of treatment.

Among men with a history of prostate cancer, the safest candidates for testosterone therapy are those with low-risk disease who have an undetectable PSA after RP. A relatively low-risk group also includes those with excellent PSA responses to radiation therapy. Until more data are available, testosterone therapy in men on active surveillance should be undertaken only with great caution. And testosterone therapy should be avoided in men with advanced or metastatic disease, and in men currently treated with androgen deprivation.

Another point to consider is that any man, with or without a history of prostate cancer, is likely to experience an increase in PSA if their baseline serum testosterone is below the saturation point. This varies from one individual to another, but the saturation point seems to be approximately 250 ng/dL. Thus, if a man begins treatment with a serum testosterone of 150 ng/dL it can be expected that his PSA will increase for the first 3 to 6 months, whereas this is less likely in a man with a baseline serum testosterone of 290 ng/dL.

For all men receiving testosterone therapy with treated or untreated prostate cancer, follow-up should be rigorous, especially in the first year of treatment. Physicians must be prepared for prostate cancer recurrence and the possibility that it may be interpreted as a result of testosterone therapy. Hematocrit and hemoglobin should be measured 2 to 4 times in the first year, then annually. PSA levels should be measured every 3 to 4 months in the first year, then biannually. Digital rectal examination should be performed 1 to 2 times in the first year, then annually. It should also be noted that for those men undergoing active surveillance, an annual prostate biopsy should be performed to ensure cancer stability. After stability has been determined, longer intervals may be suitable.

SUMMARY

There has been a revolution in thought and practice over the last 20 years regarding the relationship of testosterone and prostate cancer. The increase in the use of testosterone therapy has coincided with a growing awareness that the historical fear regarding testosterone and prostate cancer can no longer be accepted as true. Considerable evidence contradicts the notion that higher testosterone levels are associated with increased risk of developing prostate cancer, or higher grade Gleason score. The saturation model provides a satisfying explanation for why major changes in PSA are observed when a man's serum testosterone moves into or out of the castrate range. Indeed, there is now ample evidence that investigators should be more concerned about the risks of low testosterone concentrations rather than high testosterone with regard to prostate cancer. The use of testosterone therapy among men with a history of prostate cancer should no longer be considered an absolute contraindication. Scientific thought has been turned upside down over the last 20 years on the issue of testosterone therapy and prostate cancer.

REFERENCES

1. Morales A. The long and tortuous history of the discovery of testosterone and its clinical application. J Sex Med 2013;10(4):1178–83.
2. Freeman ER, Bloom DA, McGuire EJ. A brief history of testosterone. J Urol 2001;165:371–3.
3. Nieschlag E. Testosterone treatment comes of age: new options for hypogonadal men. Clin Endocrinol 2006;65:275–81.
4. Morgentaler A, Feibus A, Baum N. Testosterone and cardiovascular disease–the controversy and the facts. Postgrad Med 2014;127:159–65.
5. Aub JC. Endocrines: the use of testosterone. N Engl J Med 1940;222:877–81.
6. Huggins C, Hodges CV. The effect of castration, of estrogen and of androgen injection on serum phosphatase on metastatic carcinoma of the prostate. Cancer Res 1941;1:293–7.
7. Baillargeon J, Urban RJ, Ottenbacher KJ, et al. Trends in androgen prescribing in the United States, 2001 to 2011. JAMA Intern Med 2013;173:1465–6.

8. Zarotsky V, Huang MY, Carman W, et al. Systematic literature review of the risk factors, comorbidities, and consequences of hypogonadism in men. Andrology 2014;2:819–34.

9. Khera M, Crawford D, Morales A, et al. A new era of testosterone and prostate cancer: from physiology to clinical implications. Eur Urol 2014;65:115–23.

10. Morgentaler A. Testosterone and prostate cancer: what are the risks for middle-aged men? Urol Clin North Am 2011;38:119–24.

11. Huggins C, Stevens RE, Hodges CV. Studies on prostatic cancer: II. The effects of castration on advanced carcinoma of the prostate gland. Arch Surg 1941;43:209–23.

12. Fowler JE Jr, Whitmore WF Jr. The response of metastatic adenocarcinoma of the prostate to exogenous testosterone. J Urol 1981;126:372–5.

13. Morgentaler A. Goodbye androgen hypothesis, hello saturation model. Eur Urol 2012;62:765–7.

14. Morgentaler A. Turning conventional wisdom upside-down. Cancer 2011;117:3885–8.

15. Morgentaler A. Rapidly shifting concepts regarding androgens and prostate cancer. ScientificWorldJournal 2009;9:685–90.

16. Carson CC 3rd, Kirby R. Prostate cancer and testosterone replacement therapy-what is the risk? J Urol 2015;194(6):1527–8.

17. Morgentaler A, Bruning CO, DeWolf WC. Occult prostate cancer in men with low serum testosterone levels. JAMA 1996;276:1904–6.

18. Thompson IM, Pauler DK, Goodman PJ, et al. Prevalence of prostate cancer among men with a prostate-specific antigen level≤ 4.0 ng per milliliter. N Engl J Med 2004;350:2239–46.

19. Morgentaler A. Testosterone and prostate cancer: an historical perspective on a modern myth. Eur Urol 2006;50:935–9.

20. Endogenous Hormones and Prostate Cancer Collaborative Group, Roddam AW, Allen NE, Appleby P, et al. Endogenous sex hormones and prostate cancer: a collaborative analysis of 18 prospective studies. J Natl Cancer Inst 2008;100:170–83.

21. Muller RL, Gerber L, Moreira DM, et al. Serum testosterone and dihydrotestosterone and prostate cancer risk in the placebo arm of the reduction by dutasteride of prostate cancer events trial. Eur Urol 2012;62:757–64.

22. Rhoden EL, Morgentaler A. Risks of testosterone-replacement therapy and recommendations for monitoring. N Engl J Med 2004;350:482–92.

23. Cooper CS, Perry PJ, Sparks AE, et al. Effect of exogenous testosterone on prostate volume, serum and semen prostate specific antigen levels in healthy young men. J Urol 1998;159:441–3.

24. Bhasin S, Woodhouse L, Casaburi R, et al. Testosterone dose-response relationships in healthy young men. Am J Physiol Endocrinol Metab 2001;281:1172–81.

25. Prout GR Jr, Brewer WR. Response of men with advanced prostatic carcinoma to exogenous administration of testosterone. Cancer 1967;20:1871–8.

26. Morgentaler A, Traish AM. Shifting the paradigm of testosterone and prostate cancer: the saturation model and the limits of androgen-dependent growth. Eur Urol 2009;55:310–21.

27. Morgentaler A. Testosterone replacement therapy and prostate cancer. Urol Clin North Am 2007;34:555–63.

28. Morgentaler A, Conners WP. Testosterone therapy in men with prostate cancer: literature review, clinical experience, and recommendations. Asian J Androl 2015;17:206.

29. Ho SM, Damassa D, Kwan PW, et al. Androgen receptor levels and androgen contents in the prostate lobes of intact and testosterone-treated noble rats. J Androl 1985;6:279–90.

30. Traish AM, Williams DF, Hoffman ND, et al. Validation of the exchange assay for the measurement of androgen receptors in human and dog prostates. Prog Clin Biol Res 1988;262:145–60.

31. Marks LS, Mazer NA, Mostaghel E, et al. Effect of testosterone replacement therapy on prostate tissue in men with late-onset hypogonadism: a randomized controlled trial. JAMA 2006;296:2351–61.

32. Harman SM, Metter EJ, Tobin JD, et al. Longitudinal effects of aging on serum total and free testosterone levels in healthy men. Baltimore longitudinal study of aging. J Clin Endocrinol Metab 2001;86:724–31.

33. Kava BR. To treat or not to treat with testosterone replacement therapy: a contemporary review of management of late-onset hypogonadism and critical issues related to prostate cancer. Curr Urol Rep 2014;15:1–10.

34. Traish AM, Miner MM, Morgentaler A, et al. Testosterone deficiency. Am J Med 2011;124:578–87.

35. Calof OM, Singh AB, Lee ML, et al. Adverse events associated with testosterone replacement in middle-aged and older men: a meta-analysis of randomized, placebo-controlled trials. J Gerontol A Biol Sci Med Sci 2005;60:1451–7.

36. Shabsigh R, Crawford ED, Nehra A, et al. Testosterone therapy in hypogonadal men and potential prostate cancer risk: a systematic review. Int J Impot Res 2009;21:9–23.

37. Feneley MR, Carruthers M. Is testosterone treatment good for the prostate? Study of safety during long-term treatment. J Sex Med 2012;9:2138–49.

38. Morgentaler A. Testosterone deficiency and prostate cancer: emerging recognition of an important and troubling relationship. Eur Urol 2007;52:623–5.

39. Hoffman MA, DeWolf WC, Morgentaler A. Is low serum free testosterone a marker for high grade prostate cancer? J Urol 2000;163:8247.

40. Schatzl G, Madersbacher S, Thurridl T, et al. High-grade prostate cancer is associated with low serum testosterone levels. Prostate 2001;47:52–8.

41. Mearini L, Costantini E, Zucchi A, et al. Testosterone levels in benign prostatic hypertrophy and prostate cancer. Urol Int 2008;80:134–40.

42. García-Cruz E, Piqueras M, Huguet J, et al. Low testosterone levels are related to poor prognosis factors in men with prostate cancer prior to treatment. BJU Int 2012;110:E541–6.

43. Salonia A, Gallina A, Briganti A, et al. Preoperative hypogonadism is not an independent predictor of high-risk disease in patients undergoing radical prostatectomy. Cancer 2011;117:3953–62.

44. Yamamoto S, Yonese J, Kawakami S, et al. Preoperative serum testosterone level as an independent predictor of treatment failure following radical prostatectomy. Eur Urol 2007;52:696–701.

45. San Francisco IF, Rojas PA, DeWolf WC, et al. Low free testosterone levels predict disease reclassification in men with prostate cancer undergoing active surveillance. BJU Int 2014;114:229–35.

46. Kaplan AL, Hu JC. Use of testosterone replacement therapy in the United States and its effect on subsequent prostate cancer outcomes. Urology 2013;82:321–6.

47. Kaufman JM, Graydon RJ. Androgen replacement after curative radical prostatectomy for prostate cancer in hypogonadal men. J Urol 2004;172:920–2.

48. Agarwal PK, Oefelein MG. Testosterone replacement therapy after primary treatment for prostate cancer. J Urol 2005;173:533–6.

49. Khera M, Grober ED, Najari B, et al. Testosterone replacement therapy following radical prostatectomy. J Sex Med 2009;6:1165–70.

50. Pastuszak AW, Pearlman AM, Lai WS, et al. Testosterone replacement therapy in patients with prostate cancer after radical prostatectomy. J Urol 2013;190:639–44.

51. Sarosdy MF. Testosterone replacement for hypogonadism after treatment of early prostate cancer with brachytherapy. Cancer 2007;109:536–41.

52. Morales A, Black AM, Emerson LE. Testosterone administration to men with testosterone deficiency syndrome after external beam radiotherapy for localized prostate cancer: preliminary observations. BJU Int 2009;103:62–4.

53. Pastuszak AW, Pearlman AM, Godoy G, et al. Testosterone replacement therapy in the setting of prostate cancer treated with radiation. Int J Impot Res 2013;25:24–8.

54. Balbontin FG, Moreno SA, Bley E, et al. Long-acting testosterone injections for treatment of testosterone deficiency after brachytherapy for prostate cancer. BJU Int 2014;114:125–30.

55. Pastuszak AW, Khanna A, Badhiwala N, et al. Testosterone therapy after radiation therapy for low, intermediate, and high risk prostate cancer. J Urol 2015;194(5):1271–6.

56. Morgentaler A, Lipshultz LI, Bennett R, et al. Testosterone therapy in men with untreated prostate cancer. J Urol 2011;185:1256–60.

57. Kacker R, Mariam H, San Francisco IF, et al. Can testosterone therapy be offered to men on active surveillance for prostate cancer? Preliminary results. Asian J Androl 2016;18(1):16–20.

58. Morales A. Effect of testosterone administration to men with prostate cancer is unpredictable: a word of caution and suggestions for a registry. BJU Int 2011;107:1369–73.

Testosterone and Sexual Function

John R. Gannon, MD[a], Thomas J. Walsh, MD, MS[b],*

KEYWORDS

- Testosterone replacement therapy • Sexual dysfunction • Erectile dysfunction • Hypogonadism
- Libido • Ejaculatory function

KEY POINTS

- Sexual and erectile dysfunction are common conditions, becoming more common as men age. Hypogonadism frequently occurs concurrently with erectile dysfunction.
- The current literature seems to show a beneficial effect on sexual symptoms/function of testosterone replacement therapy (TRT) in the setting of hypogonadism.
- TRT may improve a patient's response to a phosphodiesterase inhibitor.
- Other forms of TRT seem to show a similar response, with improvement of sexual function in limited studies.

INTRODUCTION

Although "testosterone" is synonymous with "sexual function" in the lay media, the actual role of endogenous testosterone levels and the use of exogenous testosterone to predict or treat sexual dysfunction, respectively, is not clear. Testosterone levels and replacement have been linked with sexual function, specifically erection quality, libido, and ejaculatory function in a variety of studies.

To what extent serum testosterone testing is performed as a result of men presenting with complaints of sexual dysfunction is not entirely clear, despite the European Male Aging Study (EMAS), which showed a clear relationship between sexual symptoms and biochemical hypogonadism. This 2010 study conducted at 8 European centers showed a clear relationship between decreased frequency of morning erections, decreased frequency of sexual thoughts, erectile dysfunction, and serum total and free testosterone levels.[1] This study further showed an increase in symptoms correlating to declining testosterone levels.[1]

Erectile dysfunction is common and the proportion of men experiencing erectile dysfunction is expected to increase as the US population ages. It is projected that more than 35 million American men will experience erectile dysfunction, effecting up to 50% of men by age 50.[2] According to the EMAS, 30% of European men experienced erectile dysfunction; however, only 17% of these men were found to have low serum testosterone (<11 nmol/L) with proper testing.[1]

The screening for hypogonadism and subsequent testosterone treatment has continued to grow in the United States and worldwide.[3] A recent study showed this growth is not solely limited to older men, with evidence suggesting that testosterone prescriptions have nearly tripled in men in their 40s.[4] Based off estimates, testosterone prescriptions have grown from a $300 million dollar industry in 2002 to a more than $2 billion dollar industry in 2013.[5]

Penile erection is a complex process involving the interplay between penile vasculature, neural impulses, the hormonal milieu, and cognitive behavior.[6] Erectile dysfunction is among the

[a] Intermountain Urologic Institute, Intermountain Health Care, Salt Lake City, UT 84065, USA; [b] Department of Urology, University of Washington, 1959 Northeast Pacific Street, BB-1121, Box 356510, Seattle, WA, USA
* Corresponding author.
E-mail address: walsht@uw.edu

Urol Clin N Am 43 (2016) 217–222
http://dx.doi.org/10.1016/j.ucl.2016.01.008
0094-0143/16/$ – see front matter © 2016 Elsevier Inc. All rights reserved.

most common forms of sexual dysfunction, but other disorders such as decreased libido, ejaculatory disorders, and orgasmic dysfunction have a role in sexual dysfunction.[7]

Testosterone therapy has been shown to have an impact on sexual function in several studies; however, lack of standardization of sexual function assessment between studies has made their results difficult to interpret.[7] Guidelines for screening and treatment provided by multiple societies diverge regarding testosterone replacement and treatment of sexual dysfunction adding to even greater confusion among health care providers.[3,8,9]

As an example, the most recent Endocrine Society guidelines seek to differentiate androgen deficiency and erectile dysfunction as 2 independent disorders with separate etiologies that may coexist.[3] This assertion contrasts with the current European Association of Urology and other guidelines, which suggest that hypogonadism is a reversible cause of erectile dysfunction.[8,9] Regardless of this distinction, it seems that testosterone plays at least some role in the maintenance and perhaps enhancement of sexual function. This, combined with the increase in testosterone prescriptions, suggests that knowledge of the evidence both for and against the use of testosterone to treat sexual dysfunction is critical for all health care providers practicing in this clinical arena.

The goal of this article is to explore some of the current studies regarding testosterone replacement therapy (TRT) and its relation to sexual function.

PATHOPHYSIOLOGY

The impact of testosterone on male sexual function is not surprising. Several anatomic studies have revealed that androgen receptors are densely expressed in the male genital tract, the spinal nucleus, the medial preoptic area of the hypothalamus, and the bulbocavernosus muscle.[10,11]

In the central nervous system, specifically the medial preoptic area within the hypothalamus, androgens exert an influence on the release of several stimulatory neurotransmitters, including dopamine, oxytocin, and nitric oxide.[12] These neurotransmitters are not only related to sexual arousal and erection in mature subjects, but are also responsible for the control of sexual development in adolescence.[12]

In addition to their role in the central nervous system, androgens seem to be involved in the control and modulation of trabecular smooth muscle, endothelium, and fibroelastic properties of the corporal bodies.[12,13] In studies of castrated animals, the absence of circulating androgens leads to lower nitric oxide synthase activity, leading in turn to a decrease in vasodilation and erectile function. The absence of androgens may also lead to a disruption of smooth muscle relaxation and contraction in the nonadrenergic noncholinergic (NANC and α1-adrenergic pathways) associated with smooth muscle contraction within the sympathetic nervous system.[14,15]

However, not all studies have had consistent findings with regard to the role of androgens in sexual development and function. In an apparent contradiction to the findings discussed, several other animal studies have suggested that the variable regulation of the enzyme phosphodiesterase in the setting of hypogonadism may effectively compensate for the loss of androgen, thus leading to erectile preservation.[16] Importantly, these studies seem to be species dependent, and their extrapolation to human function should be guarded.[14–16]

A decrease in serum testosterone has been linked to increased connective tissue deposition within the erectile bodies and a subsequent decline in penile elasticity and overall erectile quality.[17]

ERECTILE FUNCTION

Penile erection is a complex interplay between neurologic and vascular pathways. Erectile function may be impacted negatively by vascular insults, including hypertension, hyperlipidemia, and atherosclerosis.[8] Erectile function additionally may be impacted by endocrine disorders such as diabetes and hypogonadism.[8]

A number of clinical trials have been conducted to characterize the impact of testosterone treatment on erectile function, with inconsistent findings. In an effort to consolidate the available evidence, a recent metaanalysis evaluated the effect of TRT on various aspects of sexual function, including erectile function.[7]

This metaanalysis conducted by Corona and colleagues[7] in 2014 sought to identify all randomized controlled trials comparing the effect of TRT versus placebo on sexual function (which was further broken down by cause of dysfunction). They also sought in this study to compare the effect of TRT as a supplement to phosphodiesterase inhibitors on erectile function.

Within this larger metaanalysis, 24 studies that included 1473 patients met inclusion criteria examining erectile function. To be included, studies needed to compare testosterone treatment to placebo and assess erectile function through a variety of standardized (the International

Index of Erectile Function [IIEF]) and nonstandardized methods.[7]

Overall in this analysis, testosterone treatment was associated with an improvement in erectile function with a summary risk estimate of 0.82 (95% confidence interval [CI], 0.47 to 1.17; $P = .001$); suggesting an 18% risk reduction in erectile dysfunction among those treated with testosterone.[7] A subanalysis suggested that this effect was more profound for studies whose enrollment had been limited to hypogonadal patients.[7] Studies that included either eugonadal men, or mixed (hypogonadal and eugonadal) had an effect size that was more modest.[7] When the authors used techniques aimed at reducing publication biases, they found that the association between testosterone treatment and erectile dysfunction only persisted in those patients who were hypogonadal.[7] The use of testosterone to improve sexual function was further supported by analyses of studies that used the IIEF-15. Among those studies that used the IIEF, the testosterone treatment was associated with a 3.7-point increase in the IIEF score ($P = .001$).[7]

Corona and colleagues[7] also sought to characterize the impact of study funding source on the association between testosterone treatment and erectile function. To do this, the authors divided studies into 2 groups: those that were sponsored by the pharmaceutical industry and those that were not. In these analyses, they found that the effect of androgen supplementation on erectile function was much greater among studies sponsored by pharmaceutical companies that supplied testosterone compared with studies that were not industry sponsored.[7]

The duration and timing of testosterone therapy may have a significant impact on erectile dysfunction treatment effect, and this may help to explain some of the differences in the result of metaanalyses. In other words, the effects of testosterone may be quite slow, and it may have little impact if only used for short duration.[13] A study conducted in 2011 demonstrated that it might take up to 6 months to see an impact of TRT on IIEF domains.[18] Additional studies have even suggested that an improvement of erectile function may take more than 12 months with TRT.[18,19]

Characterization of patient undergoing androgen deprivation therapy (ADT) for the treatment of prostate cancer may further help to elucidate the impact of testosterone on sexual function and more specifically erectile function. In a group of 250 men diagnosed with prostate cancer, 43% of the respondents before starting ADT had mild or no problems getting or maintaining an erection.[20] After 9 months of ADT, only 15% of the patients reported mild or no problems getting or maintaining an erection.[20] Further follow-up of these patients after cessation of ADT, showed a slow recovery back to baseline, with 43% again reporting a return of erectile function.[20]

To summarize, it seems that testosterone treatment does have a positive effect on erectile function as measured by IIEF; however, this impact is modest and limited to men with clear evidence of hypogonadism.

LIBIDO

Testosterone therapy has previously been shown to improve libido.[21,22] Sexual drive and desire is a common screening question for patients and a variation of this question is used on Androgen Deficiency in the Aging Male (ADAMs) and other screening tests.[23]

Again looking at the most recent and largest metaanalysis to date by Corona and colleagues,[7] a total of 17 studies examined libido and testosterone supplementation. These studies encompassed 1111 individuals. The overall effect of TRT on libido was varied depending on hormonal status. This result was only statistically significant in studies that enrolled either mixed (eugonadal and hypogonadal) or hypogonadal patients. The studies that enrolled the eugonadal patients had a more modest impact, which did not attain significance.[7] Interestingly again, looking at pharmaceutical sponsored studies, the effect of testosterone seemed less compared with the non–industry-sponsored studies, the opposite of the overall impact on erectile function outcomes.[7]

Further analysis by Corona and associates of the included studies revealed an inverse relation between baseline mean testosterone levels and the effect on libido in those given TRT. This effect was only statistically significant when looking at hypogonadal groups ($P = .023$).[7]

Evidence for the impact of serum testosterone on libido may again be gleaned from studies of men undergoing androgen deprivation. In the aforementioned 2012 study of men diagnosed with prostate cancer, libido was assessed before and after the initiation of ADT. At baseline, 28% had "major sexual interest."[20] Three months after initiating ADT, only 14% of men reported major sexual interest. After cessation of ADT, 19% of men reported sexual interest, suggesting that some but not all men return to baseline. Whether or not this persistent decline of libido in some men is related to serum testosterone levels is not completely clear.[20] Among men who were sexually active at the time of study enrollment, only 20% (22 patients) remained sexually active after 9 months of complete ADT.[20]

EJACULATORY FUNCTION/ORGASM

Given the high density of androgen receptors within the organs of the male genitals and ejaculatory tract, it is quite reasonable to assume that both orgasm and ejaculation may be impacted by alterations in a man's serum testosterone levels. Indeed, several studies have suggested that low serum testosterone levels may contribute to ejaculatory and orgasmic dysfunction.[5,23,24]

Testosterone is involved in the regulation of male ejaculatory reflex.[25] The aforementioned analysis by Corona and colleagues identified 10 studies that investigated the effect of testosterone treatment on orgasm. Unfortunately, most studies failed to clearly differentiate orgasm from ejaculation. Because of this limitation, we have combined these functions.

The 10 compiled studies included 677 patients. Overall, testosterone treatment was associated with improved orgasmic function.[7] A further look at these studies, including the 4 most recent, which looked at the IIEF orgasmic score as an outcome, reinforced the positive effects of testosterone supplementation and improvement in orgasmic function.[7]

Further analysis of the included 10 studies showed a statistically significant, inverse relationship between baseline testosterone levels and improvement in orgasmic function in patients treated with testosterone supplementation.[7] The mean SD difference by IIEF for orgasmic function was 1.62 ($P = .05$) when comparing testosterone supplemented groups and placebo.[7]

TESTOSTERONE SUPPLEMENTATION AND OTHER SEXUAL OUTCOMES

Of the 41 studies included in the Corona analysis, 10 studies looked at the impact of testosterone supplementation on nocturnal erections (436 patients included). Testosterone was seen to have a statistically significant positive effect ($P \leq .0001$).[7] Nocturnal erections, admittedly, do not have specific sexual impacts; however, as mentioned earlier in the discussion of the EMAS study, a decreased frequency of spontaneous morning erections have been linked to hypogonadism.[1] An improvement in nocturnal erections after TRT may be a signal of the patient responding to treatment.

Additional sexual function and health outcomes examined as part of the metaanalysis showed an improvement in the frequency of intercourse, sexual satisfaction, and overall sexual function. Looking at the mean SD for intercourse satisfaction comparing the supplemented and the placebo groups, there was a 1.503-point improvement on IIEF scores in the 4 included studies that used IIEF domains ($P = .017$).[7]

TESTOSTERONE SUPPLEMENTATION AND PHOSPHODIESTERASE TYPE 5 INHIBITORS

Given the common age of incidence for hypogonadism and erectile dysfunction these conditions frequently coexist in aging men.[1,8] The initial paradigm of treatment was to use testosterone therapy as an adjuvant therapy in men who had failed to respond to phosphodiesterase type 5 inhibitors alone.[22] This so-called salvage therapy sought to alleviate symptoms of hypogonadism and erectile function simultaneously and was examined in numerous studies.[21,22] Other studies have instead looked at 'combination therapy' as an additive approach for the optimization of sexual and erectile function. The analysis of data from the Tadafil and Testosterone Supplementation (TADTEST) showed a variable response to salvage therapy, with between 32% and 100% of patients who initially failed phosphodiesterase type 5 inhibitors therapy having an improvement in erectile function when given testosterone gel supplementation.[22] More recent studies have questioned combination therapy, and whether erectile function responds completely to phosphodiesterase type 5 inhibitors therapy, although this remains an active area of research.

The role of TRT in hypogonadal men with symptoms beyond erectile dysfunction; decreased libido, orgasm dysfunction, and so on, seems to be beneficial.[1,7] Similarly, erectile dysfunction with a clear etiology not attributed to hypogonadism requires therapy beyond testosterone replacement.

NONTESTOSTERONE SUPPLEMENTATION AND SEXUAL FUNCTION

Additional studies not using traditional testosterone supplementation, although limited, have been conducted. Rather than using direct replacement like TRT these studies instead used hypothalamic–pituitary–gonadal stimulation to cause an endogenous increase in serum testosterone, via clomiphene citrate or hCG. In 1995, Guay and colleagues[26] demonstrated that using clomiphene to normalize serum testosterone levels led to 39% of men having an improved, satisfactory erectile response. Further, an older study looking at human chorionic gonadotropin use, showed that approximately one-half of men given human chorionic gonadotropin to attain eugonadal levels had an improvement in the frequency of sexual activity.[27]

SUMMARY

Testosterone and sexual function are related. Baseline testosterone levels and the role of TRT have been used for identification and the treatment of decreased energy, erectile dysfunction, and decreased libido.[1,8] Current evidence suggests that TRT may improve sexual dysfunction. Sexual dysfunction from erectile dysfunction, decreased libido, and ejaculatory dysfunction in men who are hypogonadal, mixed, or eugonadal have all been examined through numerous studies. The most recent large analysis showed an overall improvement in sexual function outcomes in men treated with TRT.

Sexual function is a complex interplay of neuroendocrine and physiologic factors. It is clear from evidence in recent studies that men with documented hypogonadism benefit more from TRT than patients who are eugonadal in the treatment of sexual dysfunction. Despite evidence of these benefits, it remains prudent to discuss with patients the risks and benefits of TRT so that the patient can make an informed clinical decision.

REFERENCES

1. Wu FC, Tajar A, Beynon JM, et al. Identification of late-onset hypogonadism in middle-aged and elderly men. N Engl J Med 2010;363:123–35.

2. Aytac IA, Araujo AB, Johannes CB, et al. Socioeconomic factors and incidence of erectile dysfunction: findings of the longitudinal Massachusetts male aging study. Soc Sci Med 2000;51(5):771–8.

3. Bhasin S, Cunningham GR, Hayes FJ, et al, Task Force Endocrine Society. Testosterone therapy in men with androgen deficiency syndromes: an endocrine society clinical practice guidelines. J Clin Endocrinol Metab 2010;95:2536–59.

4. Baillargeon J, Urban RJ, Ottenbacher KJ, et al. Trends in androgen prescribing in the United States, 2001 to 2011. JAMA Intern Med 2013;173:1465.

5. Statista. Annual testosterone drug revenue in the U.S. in 2013 and 2018 (in billion U.S. dollars). Available at: www.statista.com/statistics/320301/predicted-annual-testosterone-drug-revenues-in-the-us/. Accessed July 3, 2015.

6. Steidle C, Schwartz S, Jacoby K, et al. AA2500 testosterone gel normalizes androgen levels in aging males with improvements in body composition and sexual function. J Clin Endocrinol Metab 2003;88(6):2673–81.

7. Corona G, Isidori A, Buvat J, et al. Testosterone supplementation and sexual function: a meta-analysis study. J Sex Med 2014;11:1577–92.

8. Wein AJ, editor in chief. In: Campbell MF, Wein AJ, Kavoussi LR, editors. Campbell-Walsh urology. Philadelphia: W.B. Saunders; 2010.

9. O'Connor DB, Lee DM, Corona G, et al. The relationships between sex hormones and sexual function in middle-aged and older European men. J Clin Endocrinol Metab 2011;96:1577–87.

10. Corona G, Mannucci E, Petrone L, et al. Pyschobiological correlates of delayed ejaculation in male patients with sexual dysfunctions. J Androl 2006;27(3):453–8.

11. Lewis RW, Mills TM. Effect of androgen on penile tissue. Endocrine 2004;23:101–5.

12. Hull EM, Lorrain DS, Du J, et al. Hormone-neurotransmitter interactions in the control of sexual behavior. Behav Brain Res 1999;105:105–16.

13. Isidori AM, Buvat J, Corona G, et al. A critical analysis of the role of testosterone in erectile function: from pathophysiology to treatment-a systemic review. Eur Urol 2014;65:99–112.

14. Lugg J, Ng C, Rajfer J, et al. Cavernosal nerve stimulation in the rat reverses castration-induced decrease in penile NOS activity. Am J Physiol 1996;271:E354–61.

15. Giuliano F, Rampin O, Schirar A, et al. Autonomic control of penile erection: modulation by testosterone in the rat. J Neuroendocrinol 1993;5:677–83.

16. Andric SA, Janjic MM, Stojkov NJ, et al. Testosterone-induced modulation of nitric oxide-cGMP signaling pathway and androgenesis in the rat Leydig cells. Biol Reprod 2010;83:434–42.

17. Traish AM, Park K, Dhir V, et al. Effects of castration and androgen replacement on erectile function in a rabbit model. Endocrinology 1999;140:1861–8.

18. Saad F, Aversa A, Isidori AM, et al. Onset of effects of testosterone treatment and time span until maximum effects are achieved. Eur J Endocrinol 2011;165:675–85.

19. Hackett G, Cole N, Bhartia M, et al. Testosterone replacement therapy with long-acting testosterone undecanoate improves sexual function and quality-of-life parameters vs. placebo in a population of men with type 2 diabetes. J Sex Med 2013;10:1612–27.

20. Ng E, Woo HH, Turner S, et al. The influence of testosterone suppression and recovery on sexual function in men with prostate cancer: observations from a prospective study in men undergoing intermittent androgen suppression. J Urol 2012;197:2162–7.

21. Shamloul R, Ghanem H, Fahmy I, et al. Testosterone therapy can enhance erectile function response to sildenafil in patients with PADAM: a pilot study. J Sex Med 2005;2:559–64.

22. Buvat J, Montorsi F, Maggi M, et al. Hypogonadal men nonresponders to the PDE5 inhibitor tadalafil benefit from normalization of testosterone levels with a 1% hydroalcoholic testosterone gel in the treatment of erectile dysfunction (TADTEST study). J Sex Med 2011;8:284–93.

23. Mohamed O, Freundlich RE, Dakik HK, et al. The quantitative ADAM questionnaire: a new toll in

quantifying the severity of hypogonadism. Int J Impot Res 2010;22(1):20–4.

24. Spitzer M, Basaria S, Travison TG, et al. Effect of testosterone replacement on response to sildenafil citrate in men with erectile dysfunction: a parallel, randomized trial. Ann Intern Med 2012; 157:681–91.

25. Corona G, Jannini EA, Vignozzi L, et al. The hormonal control of ejaculation. Nat Rev Urol 2012;9:508–19.

26. Guay AT, Bansal S, Heatley GJ. Effect of raising endogenous testosterone levels in impotent men with secondary hypogonadism: double blind placebo-controlled trial with clomiphene citrate. J Clin Endocrinol Metab 1995;80:3546–52.

27. Buvat J, Lemaire A, Buvat-Herbaut M. Human chorionic gonadotropin treatment of nonorganic erectile failure and lack of sexual desire: a double-blind study. Urology 1987;30:216–9.

Testosterone and Varicocele

Russell P. Hayden, MD, Cigdem Tanrikut, MD*

KEYWORDS

- Varicocele • Hypogonadism • Leydig cell • Erectile dysfunction • Testosterone • Steroidogenesis
- Androgen receptor • Varicocelectomy

KEY POINTS

- A multitude of studies suggests an adverse effect of varicocele on Leydig cell function.
- Men with lower preoperative serum testosterone levels have greater improvements in postvaricocelectomy testosterone levels as compared with eugonadal men.
- The pathophysiology of varicocele-mediated hypogonadism is poorly understood and remains an area of continued investigation.

INTRODUCTION

A varicocele is an aberrant dilation of the pampiniform plexus, the network of veins draining the testis. It is a common entity with a prevalence of 10% to 20% in the general population.[1,2] Most varicoceles are asymptomatic and have an inconsequential impact on the individual's testicular function. However, a small subset of men will present with infertility, orchialgia, or ipsilateral testicular hypotrophy, which serve as common indications for varicocelectomy.[3,4]

Traditionally, varicocele has been characterized by its impact on spermatogenesis via local effects on Sertoli and germ cells. It has become more evident, however, that varicocele presents a pantesticular insult. Leydig cell dysfunction is now a recognized potential consequence of varicocele and appears to be a reversible phenomenon with varicocelectomy.[5] Multiple mechanisms for decreased androgen production have been proposed, likely reflecting a multifactorial process. Nevertheless, the pathophysiology of varicocele-mediated Leydig cell dysfunction, as with the cause of the varicocele's link to subfertility, remains an area of ongoing research.

CLINICAL DATA

Early Evidence

Initial reports exploring the possible impact of varicocele on testosterone production were limited by retrospective design, small cohorts, and selection bias.[6-9] In addition, certain subsets of men will have worse Leydig cell function than others, an issue that may have limited studies that had permissive inclusion criteria. Comhaire and Vermeulen[10] published one of the earliest reports documenting normalization of total testosterone levels in men undergoing varicocelectomy. In their small cohort of 33 men presenting with a clinical varicocele, 10 of the men had low serum testosterone levels (mean <400 ng/dL) and concomitant erectile dysfunction, both of which improved after varicocele repair. This initial account precipitated several other analyses of cohorts of men who presented with infertility and concurrent varicocele. In 1978, Rodriguez-Rigau and colleagues[11] expanded on Comhaire's work and analyzed a group with palpable varicoceles who also underwent testicular biopsy as part of their fertility evaluation. All subjects had serum testosterone levels in the normal range, albeit subjects with

Disclosures: None.
Funding: None.
Department of Urology, Massachusetts General Hospital, 55 Fruit Street, GRB 1102, Boston, MA 02114, USA
* Corresponding author. MGH Fertility Center, 55 Fruit Street, YAW 10A, Boston, MA 02114.
E-mail address: ctanrikut@mgh.harvard.edu

Urol Clin N Am 43 (2016) 223–232
http://dx.doi.org/10.1016/j.ucl.2016.01.009

bilateral varicoceles typically had lower levels than those with unilateral varicoceles. Histopathologic assessment of the biopsy samples revealed diminished Leydig cell counts that were especially pronounced in men with concomitant oligospermia. In addition, they identified an abnormal testosterone-to-luteinizing hormone (LH) ratio in men with worse spermatogenesis. From these data, they postulated that varicocele affects all functions and cell lines of the testis.

Multiple small series followed that refuted the concept that varicoceles result in decreased testosterone synthesis.[6,7,12–14] A study by Pirke and colleagues[7] found normal testosterone levels among 21 subjects who presented with varicocele, a result mirrored by Weiss and colleagues,[8] who reported on a cohort of 16 men with accompanying hypospermatogenesis. A contemporaneous analysis by Pasqualini and colleagues[6] also documented normal testosterone levels in a group of 17 patients; however, their data did demonstrate elevated LH levels, leading to the conclusion that men with varicoceles can have normal androgen levels via compensated LH production.

These early conflicting accounts were offset by progressively larger cohorts that offered higher-quality evidence. In 1984, Ando and colleagues[15] published their account of 108 infertile men with varicocele compared against 46 infertile men without varicocele. Those men with varicocele had significantly lower testosterone levels regardless of degree of oligospermia. The group also documented worse testosterone concentrations for those men who had their varicoceles for longer lengths of time. This finding suggested that varicocele imposes progressive negative impacts on both spermatogenesis and Leydig cell function.[15,16] Subsequently, in 1995, Su and colleagues[17] reviewed their experience in men undergoing varicocelectomy. In a group of 53 patients, they found a statistically significant increase of serum testosterone from a mean preoperative level of 319 ng/dL to a postoperative value of 409 ng/dL. Their analysis also demonstrated an inverse relationship between preoperative testosterone concentration and anticipated postoperative testosterone increase. This finding raised the possibility that some men, especially those with poorer preoperative Leydig cell function, may disproportionately be affected by their varicocele and may have meaningful improvements in testosterone after varicocelectomy.

Contemporary Evidence

The work of Su and colleagues[17] was further bolstered by multiple studies that documented improved testosterone levels following varicocele repair (**Table 1**). Cayan and colleagues[18] followed 78 men who underwent varicocelectomy, quoting an improvement of mean serum testosterone from 563 to 837 ng/dL. In a similar cohort, Gat and colleagues[19] found significant improvements of total and free testosterone following gonadal vein embolization, suggesting that the positive effect of varicocele repair may not be sensitive to mode of treatment.

Despite these compelling data, many investigators continued to find insignificant improvements of testosterone following varicocelectomy.[20–22] Rodriguez-Peña and colleagues[22] reported a group of 202 patients with grade II or III varicoceles. Their results demonstrated a mean testosterone increase of 61 ng/dL, although the finding did not reach statistical significance. In another large series by Al-Ali colleagues[23] in which 1111 men had presented for infertility evaluation, the presence of grade III varicoceles was actually associated with higher testosterone levels. These conflicting reports were ultimately contextualized by Hsiao and colleagues[24] in 2011. In this series, 106 men underwent hormonal evaluation before and after varicocelectomy similar to previous study designs. However, Hsiao and colleagues stratified their cohort into men with eugonadal testosterone levels and biochemical hypogonadism ($\geq$ or <400 ng/dL, respectively). As was the case with Su's initial finding in 1996, men with lower initial serum testosterone experienced far greater increases in their androgen levels as opposed to the eugonadal individuals.[17] Many of the studies that did not find significant improvements of serum testosterone following varicocele repair had cohorts characterized by normal preoperative testosterone levels (ie, greater than 400 ng/dL).[20–22,25] For instance, the study subjects of Rodriguez-Peña and colleagues[22] had a mean preoperative testosterone level of 648 ng/dL. The cohort of Pierik and colleagues[20] was also eugonadal in 90% of the cases.

Several studies have corroborated Hsiao's finding.[24] Tanrikut and colleagues[26] examined a large series of 325 men who had undergone varicocelectomy for infertility and contrasted them against 510 men who presented for vasectomy. The varicocele group had significantly lower serum testosterone levels than control subjects. Of the 200 men in whom both preoperative and postoperative hormonal profiles were available, a mean testosterone increase of 96 ng/dL was demonstrated. They found that 79% of the men with initial testosterone levels less than 300 ng/dL had normal testosterone concentrations following varicocelectomy. A similar study

Table 1
Significant studies documenting baseline and postvaricocele repair testosterone levels

First Author, Year	Study Design	Number Treated for Varicocele	Baseline Testosterone (ng/dL)	Postoperative Testosterone (ng/dL)	Change (ng/dL)	P Value
Shabana et al,[30] 2015	Prospective	123	385	447	62	.0001
Ahmed et al,[29] 2015	Prospective	73	331	357	26	.001
Abdel-Meguid et al,[28] 2014	Prospective	66	347	392	45	.0001
Hsiao et al,[68] 2013	Retrospective	78	308	417	109	.0001
Hsiao et al,[24] 2011	Retrospective	—	—	—	—	—
Age <30		31	NA	NA	93	.03
Age 30–39		55	NA	NA	59	.02
Age >40		28	NA	NA	73	.001
Sathya Srini & Belur Veerachari,[27] 2011	Prospective	100	177	301	124	.001
Tanrikut et al,[26] 2011	Retrospective	200	358	454	96	.001
Zohdy et al,[31] 2011	Prospective	103	379	450	71	.0001
Resorlu et al,[21] 2010	Retrospective	—	—	—	—	—
Age 18–25		35	275	297	22	>.05
Age 26–35		43	290	306	16	>.05
Age >36		18	274	291	17	>.05
Rodriguez-Peña et al,[22] 2009	Retrospective	202	648	709	61	>.05
Ozden et al,[69] 2008	Prospective	30	660	720	60	.1
Di Bisceglie et al,[25] 2007	Retrospective	38	650	660	10	.9
Hurtado de Catalfo et al,[51] 2007	Retrospective	36	298	382	84	NA
Gat et al,[19] 2004	Retrospective	83	348	497	149	.001
Fujisawa et al,[70] 2001	Retrospective	52	460	470	10	>.05
Pierik et al,[20] 2001	Retrospective	30	542	571	29	>.05
Cayan et al,[18] 1999	Retrospective	78	563	837	274	.01
Su et al,[17] 1995	Retrospective	53	319	409	90	.001

by Sathya Srini and Belur Veerachari[27] included only those infertile men with varicoceles and preoperative testosterone levels less than 280 ng/dL. Half of their cohort underwent varicocele repair, whereas the other half chose to proceed directly to assisted reproduction. The surgical group had postoperative normalization of their testosterone levels in 78% of cases, whereas only 16% of control subjects had normalization over the same time span. The most dramatic results that expanded on the observations of Su and colleagues and Hsiao and colleagues were published by Abdel-Meguid and colleagues in 2014.[28] In this well-powered study, only those men with pre-existing biochemical hypogonadism (<300 ng/dL) had a significant increase of testosterone level following varicocele repair. This

subgroup of patients had a mean testosterone increment of 93.7 ng/dL as opposed to 8.6 ng/dL in eugonadal men.

The quality of evidence linking varicocelectomy to increased androgen production has continued to improve with time. A summative meta-analysis by Li and colleagues[5] incorporated 9 studies with a total of 814 patients. The pooled data yielded a mean testosterone increase of 97.5 ng/dL following varicocele repair. More recently, investigators have used prospective study designs. Ahmed and colleagues[29] enrolled 129 patients and followed them to 6 months after varicocelectomy. The mean testosterone concentration increased from 331 to 357 ng/dL. In 2015, Shabana and colleagues[30] published a similar prospective study with a cohort of 123 patients noting mean prevaricocelectomy and postvaricocelectomy values of 385 and 447 ng/dL, respectively. These 2 studies complemented other prospective trials that demonstrated similar results[28,31].

The preponderance of evidence supports the link between varicocele and diminished Leydig cell function in man. Unfortunately, one must rely on a set of publications that may be flawed by selection bias, given the impracticality of conducting a randomized trial in patients who often present with infertility and desire varicocelectomy. Even when viewed from this lens, one cannot ignore the number of well-fashioned studies that include relatively large numbers of subjects.[24,26,28–31] Although a great deal of work has thus established the link between varicocele and decreased androgen production, the pathophysiologic principles that result in this association have yet to be identified.

PATHOPHYSIOLOGY OF LEYDIG CELL DYSFUNCTION
Human Studies

The mechanisms proposed to explain how varicoceles may adversely affect Leydig cells closely parallel the classic theories of varicocele-mediated infertility. It is likely that the Leydig cell reacts similarly to Sertoli and germ cells when exposed to hypoxia, hyperthermia, gonadal/adrenal toxins, and oxidative stress, all of which may be derived from impaired venous drainage. Some investigators have even proposed that impaired testosterone secretion is causal to subsequent hypospermatogenesis.[8,11,30,32,33] Others have submitted evidence that deficient spermatogenesis and Leydig cell dysfunction are independent processes that share common upstream causal events.[6,7,34–36] Although both viewpoints seem to be at odds, as with most biologic systems, it is likely that decreased testosterone synthesis and impaired sperm production share both a direct causal link and common precursor mechanisms.

Early human studies concentrated on the hypothalamic-pituitary-testis (HPT) axis in men with concomitant varicocele and subfertility. Hudson and colleagues[37] used a bolus of gonadotropin-releasing hormone (GnRH) to study the HPT axis in men with and without varicocele. They repeated the protocol in subjects who underwent varicocele repair.[32] Their data demonstrated that men with varicoceles typically have an excessive release of LH in response to the GnRH bolus as compared with normal individuals. In addition, 63% of men who had varicocelectomy experienced normalization of their serum testosterone response to the GnRH stimulation. The

investigators concluded that varicoceles result in a global testicular defect as evidenced by derangement of the HPT axis, which may be reversible in some men who undergo varicocele repair. The early work by Hudson was further developed by Ando and colleagues,[15] who followed an expanded hormonal profile within peripheral and spermatic cord veins.[38] These investigators also used a GnRH bolus to probe the HPT axis of subjects with varicocele. Their results corroborated the tendency of diminished testosterone secretion in varicocele-afflicted men when compared with controls. The broader analysis of the steroidogenic pathway enabled Ando and his colleagues to evaluate for potential enzymatic block or dysfunction. In men with varicocele, they demonstrated excessive amounts of 17-hydroxyprogesterone and a markedly elevated 17-hydroxyprogesterone:testosterone ratio (**Fig. 1**). These data indicate a possible defect at the level of 17,20-lyase and, to a lesser degree, 17α-hydroxylase. It has been proposed that these enzymes are particularly sensitive to hyperthermia, a known consequence of varicocele formation.[9,18,39,40] A subsequent study by Osuna and colleagues[14] confirmed similar endocrine results in an adolescent cohort with varicocele and preserved total testosterone.

Unlike the GnRH studies, results from human chorionic gonadotropin (HCG)-mediated stimulation of the Leydig cells have led to conflicting results. Pirke and colleagues[7] studied 21 patients who underwent a single injection of HCG. They found similar baseline levels of testosterone excretion in men with varicoceles as compared with controls. Post-HCG testosterone concentrations increased markedly, which indicated that Leydig

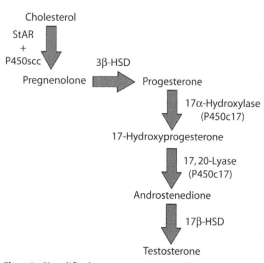

Fig. 1. Simplified testosterone synthesis pathway. HSD, hydroxysteroid dehydrogenase.

cell function was adequate. They concluded that Leydig cell function is normal in the varicocele population. The results of Pirke were in direct conflict with a contemporaneous study by Scholler and colleagues,[41] who used a larger HCG bolus and measured an expanded hormonal profile over several time points. A blunted testosterone response was observed as compared with controls. Similar to Ando and colleagues,[15] Scholler and colleagues observed significant elevations of 17-hydroxyprogesterone.[38] Again, this indicated a possible impairment at the level of 17,20-lyase. When comparing the methods of Pirke versus those of Scholler, it becomes apparent that HCG stimulation may require higher doses in conjunction with time-sensitive measurements.

Other investigators have attempted to clarify the varicocele's effect on Leydig cells through quantitative and qualitative observations of testicular biopsy samples. Sirvent and colleagues[42] analyzed testis biopsies from 31 men who presented with varicocele. In addition to the pathognomonic atrophy of seminiferous tubules, they observed multiple changes in the characteristics of the Leydig cell population. Interestingly, men with varicoceles had Leydig cell hyperplasia. Ultrastructural analysis revealed further abnormalities, most notably vacuolization of the cytoplasm. Sirvent went further by functionally testing the expanded population of Leydig cells with the peroxidase-antiperoxidase method, which demonstrated a decreased number of cells expressing testosterone. It is remarkable that all men in their cohort had normal peripheral levels of LH and testosterone, leading the investigators to conclude that men with varicoceles must compensate via Leydig cell hyperplasia in order to remain eugonadal. In a similar study by Francavilla and colleagues,[43] 23 testicular biopsies from men afflicted with varicocele were evaluated. They too observed Leydig cell hyperplasia, which correlated with the severity of concomitant oligospermia. Both Sirvent and Francavilla contradicted an earlier study by Weiss and colleagues, who did not observe Leydig cell hyperplasia in a cohort of men with severe hypospermatogenesis.[44] This discrepancy may be a result of the narrower inclusion criteria of Weiss in conjunction with an underpowered design (n = 16). A notable finding of all 3 studies was uniform changes to the Leydig cell populations in both testes despite most of the subjects presenting with unilateral varicocele.[42–44] These data further support the notion that unilateral varicoceles result in bilateral testicular effects.[40,45]

A follow-up study by Weiss and colleagues[8] tested the in vitro ability of biopsied Leydig cells to produce testosterone. Although their subjects had normal LH and serum testosterone levels, deficient synthetic activity was observed for the in vitro samples. They hypothesized that men presenting with concurrent varicocele and oligospermia may have diminished intratesticular testosterone levels that drive hypospermatogenesis, given that an adequate concentration of intratesticular testosterone is necessary for sperm production.[46,47] One notable study by Pasqualini and colleagues[6] directly measured intratesticular testosterone in 17 subjects with varicocele. They found a mean testosterone concentration of 906 ng/g of testicular tissue, which corresponds to a high-normal value; most patients within Pasqualini's study had normal serum testosterone levels as well. As previously discussed, Hsiao and colleagues[24] found that principally men with pre-existing hypogonadism had appreciable improvements from varicocelectomy. Pasqualini's cohort underrepresented the subpopulation of individuals who seem to have significant varicocele-mediated Leydig cell dysfunction. No adequately powered human studies exist that evaluate intratesticular testosterone in strictly hypogonadal men with varicocele.

The early work that attempted to elucidate the mechanisms behind varicocele and decreased testosterone secretion hypothesized that testicular hyperthermia is the keystone of impaired steroidogenesis. However, recent studies have begun to delve into other causes of Leydig cell impairment. It is known that higher scrotal temperatures result in elevated reactive oxygen species (ROS), which may serve as the next causal step in hormonal dysregulation secondary to varicocele.[34] Multiple studies have already connected subfertility from varicoceles with elevated oxidative stress.[48–50] Similar data are emerging for a link to Leydig cell dysfunction. Hurtado de Catalfo and colleagues[51] compared levels of antioxidants and serum testosterone in 36 infertile men undergoing varicocelectomy against 33 controls. Their data demonstrated decreased levels of antioxidants in men with varicocele, both in semen and in venous blood, which normalized following varicocele repair. Serum testosterone concentrations also significantly improved in parallel with the antioxidant levels. Although compelling, one must assume confounding could have tainted the results as the subjects originally presented with infertility, a condition for which an association with ROS has already been documented. To sufficiently control for such confounders, researchers turned to animal studies to better evaluate the negative effects of varicocele.

Animal Studies

Animal models have been used in an attempt to specify the pathophysiologic interplay between varicocele and androgen production. Multiple groups have recapitulated a dilated pampiniform plexus with subsequent development of infertility and decreased steroidogenesis in various animal models.[52–58] These studies afford a control group that is often subjected to sham procedures, thereby providing a strong level of evidence. One of the first notable investigations that addressed androgen production in the setting of varicocele was conducted by Rajfer and colleagues.[52] They used an established rat model to demonstrate that intratesticular testosterone decreased by nearly half at 2 weeks after varicocele creation. Similar to the work of Ando and colleagues[15] in humans, Rajfer found significant impairment of the 17,20-lyase and 17α-hydroxylase enzymes. Rajfer and colleagues also postulated that elevated scrotal temperatures directly impact the kinetics of both enzymes.

Multiple other studies have also found a significant decline of intratesticular testosterone in rodent models even though the same process has been difficult to establish in humans.[6] Ghosh and York[58] demonstrated that both serum and intratesticular testosterone concentrations diminished with a surgically induced varicocele. Zheng and colleagues[53] attempted a similar protocol, but with differing lengths of time until the testis was extirpated for analysis. They demonstrated a progressive and continuous decline of intratesticular testosterone with longer varicocele durations.

One novel mechanism for the progressive drop of intratesticular testosterone was proposed by Sweeney and colleagues.[33] They found that 90% of the additional venous pressure caused by a varicocele is transmitted to the postcapillary venule within the hamster testis. Intratesticular testosterone is typically carried to its targets through the interstitial fluid.[59] Disruption of the precapillary and postcapillary pressures will disrupt the balance that drives capillary filtration. Added venule pressure results in greater capillary filtration, possibly with an accompanying washout of intratesticular testosterone. Such a local decrease of testosterone concentration may also affect the epididymis and its functions on sperm maturation, especially in regards to motility.[11,60]

A separate mechanism from that of Sweeney's was put forth by the results of Luo and colleagues.[55] They found that along with the drop of intratesticular testosterone, messenger RNA for the steroidogenic acute regulatory protein (StAR) was significantly decreased. StAR serves as a transporter for cholesterol across the mitochondrial membrane and is the first and rate-limiting step of steroid synthesis. A follow-up study by Diemer and colleagues[35] used hydrogen peroxide to induce oxidative stress and measured perturbations of the StAR protein. They found that both expression and activity of StAR were exquisitely sensitive to oxidative stress, and that the effect reverses following removal of the insult. The data of Diemer and colleagues mirror the results of an older study that also found diminished transport of cholesterol into the mitochondria during periods of elevated oxidative stress.[36]

Leydig cells appear particularly vulnerable to ROS, especially given that they reside in proximity to interstitial macrophages: one of the principal contributors to endogenous ROS.[35] However, varicoceles may also affect intratesticular signaling through the androgen receptor. Soares and colleagues[61] measured the transcription and expression of estrogen and androgen receptors following varicocele induction in rats. They found normal amounts of androgen receptor transcription; however, protein levels of the androgen receptor were significantly decreased. Not only do varicoceles appear to inhibit steroidogenesis, but also they may inhibit the cell's ability to receive the androgen signal within the testis. Analogous results have been corroborated in man.[60] The results of Soares and colleagues reiterate the multifactorial nature of varicocele pathophysiology.

VARICOCELECTOMY FOR HYPOGONADISM— CLINICAL SIGNIFICANCE

Hypogonadism remains a controversial indication for varicocele repair.[4] It is clear from both animal and human studies that varicocele impedes testosterone synthesis and androgen signaling at multiple levels.[8,15,34,61] In addition, it is now evident that varicocelectomy improves serum testosterone levels, with the largest benefit to those who have lower testosterone concentrations preoperatively.[24,26,28] The expected improvement of serum testosterone has been shown to be approximately 90 ng/dL in the most favorable studies.[24,26,28] It remains vague, however, whether the modest improvements of serum testosterone after varicocelectomy result in clinically meaningful improvement of hypogonadal symptoms.

Most studies that evaluate improvement of symptomatic hypogonadism following varicocelectomy concentrate on sexual health. One of the first descriptions of a positive impact on sexual dysfunction was published by Comhaire and Vermeulen[10] in 1975. In this small study, 10 subjects endorsed erectile dysfunction, and the majority recovered erectile function following varicocele repair. Another report by Younes,[62] which followed a cohort of 48 men, reported an improvement in sexual activity of 50% to 75%. Unfortunately, the results of these 2 studies are difficult to interpret given that both suffer from small cohorts and vague endpoints.

A large retrospective review by Lotti and colleagues[63] examined a consecutive series of 2448 men who presented for sexual complaints. Their careful analysis found that premature ejaculation was the only symptom associated with the presence of varicocele. Although erectile dysfunction tended to occur more commonly in those with varicocele, this did not reach statistical significance. Zohdy and colleagues[31] subsequently published a prospective study of infertile men with varicocele in which erectile dysfunction, measured via the International Index of Erectile Function (IIEF-5), served as one of the primary endpoints. In their cohort of 141 patients, they found that those who elected for varicocelectomy had a score improvement on their IIEF-5 from 17.1 to 19.7. In a similar study, Sathya Srini and Belur Veerachari[27] also reported a small improvement in erectile dysfunction in their cohort of 200 men. Of note, the presenting complaint in both cohorts was infertility. Consequently, the data must be viewed cautiously given the complex interplay between infertility and sexual dysfunction.[64,65] A subsequent population-based study that did not recruit from fertility clinics, although limited by its case-control design and reliance on claims data, found an odds ratio of 3.09 for erectile dysfunction when comparing those with and without a varicocele.[66]

Overall, the evidence linking varicoceles to erectile dysfunction is flawed. In order to maximize any possible benefit, an attempted varicocele repair must strive for maximum improvement of postoperative testosterone. In this regard, technique may prove meaningful based on the results of Zheng and colleagues.[56] The investigators of this study evaluated artery-preserving versus artery-ligating varicocelectomy in an animal model. Their results demonstrated substantially lower values of intratesticular testosterone when the testicular artery was not spared. This enlightening result can be extrapolated to humans in which optical magnification is not always used during varicocele repair, perhaps inadvertently placing the patient's testicular artery at risk.[67] Ideally, practitioners who offer varicocelectomy should make every effort to spare the testicular artery. Even in this setting, however, the small improvements of serum testosterone concentration may not result in subjective improvement. The hypogonadal symptoms with which patients present are often multifactorial, and so caution should be used when setting postoperative expectations.

SUMMARY

Varicocele causes a global negative impact on testis function, including the paracrine and endocrine functions of the Leydig cell. The relationship between varicocele and diminished androgen levels is now well-established and appears to be reversible with varicocele repair. Men with pre-existing hypogonadism gain greater benefit from varicocelectomy in terms of postoperative improvement of their hormonal parameters. Nonetheless, hypogonadism remains a controversial indication for varicocelectomy. The modest improvement of postoperative testosterone concentration may not manifest clinically, and patients must be carefully counseled to maintain appropriate expectations. Last, multiple mechanisms linking vein dilation to impaired testosterone synthesis, secretion, and signaling appear to exist. Further study is required to clarify the multifactorial pathophysiology of varicocele-mediated Leydig cell dysfunction.

REFERENCES

1. The influence of varicocele on parameters of fertility in a large group of men presenting to infertility clinics. World Health Organization. Fertil Steril 1992;57(6):1289–93.
2. Masson P, Brannigan RE. The varicocele. Urol Clin North Am 2014;41(1):129–44.
3. Nagler HM, Grotas AB. Varicocele. In: Lipshultz LI, Howards SS, Niederberger CS, editors. Infertility in the male. 4th edition. Cambridge (United Kingdom): Cambridge University Press; 2009. p. 331–61.
4. Schlegel PN, Goldstein M. Alternate indications for varicocele repair: non-obstructive azoospermia, pain, androgen deficiency and progressive testicular dysfunction. Fertil Steril 2011;96(6):1288–93.
5. Li F, Yue H, Yamaguchi K, et al. Effect of surgical repair on testosterone production in infertile men with varicocele: a meta-analysis. Int J Urol 2012; 19(2):149–54.
6. Pasqualini T, Chemes H, Coco R, et al. Testicular function in varicocele. Int J Androl 1980;3(6):679–91.
7. Pirke KM, Vogt HJ, Sintermann R, et al. Testosterone in peripheral plasma, spermatic vein and in testicular tissue under basal conditions and after HCG-stimulation in patients with varicocele. Andrologia 1983;15(6):637–41.
8. Weiss DB, Rodrigues-Rigau L, Smith KD, et al. Leydig cell density and function and their relation to gonadotropins in infertile oligospermic men with varicocele. Isr J Med Sci 1979;15(7):556–63.

9. Ishikawa T, Fujisawa M. Varicocele ligation on free testosterone levels in infertile men with varicocele. Arch Androl 2004;50(6):443–8.

10. Comhaire F, Vermeulen A. Plasma testosterone in patients with varicocele and sexual inadequacy. J Clin Endocrinol Metab 1975;40(5):824–9.

11. Rodriguez-Rigau LJ, Weiss DB, Zukerman Z, et al. A possible mechanism for the detrimental effect of varicocele on testicular function in man. Fertil Steril 1978;30(5):577–85.

12. Cantatore C, Capuano P, Cobuzzi I, et al. Semen quality and hormonal levels in infertile patients with varicocele. Arch Ital Urol Androl 2010;82(4):291–3.

13. Canales B, Zapzalka D, Ercole C, et al. Prevalence and effect of varicoceles in an elderly population. Urology 2005;66(3):627–31.

14. Osuna JA, Lozano JR, Cruz I, et al. Pituitary and testicular function in adolescents with varicocele. Arch Androl 1999;43(3):183–8.

15. Ando S, Giacchetto C, Colpi G, et al. Physiopathologic aspects of Leydig cell function in varicocele patients. J Androl 1984;5(3):163–70.

16. Gorelick JI, Goldstein M. Loss of fertility in men with varicocele. Fertil Steril 1993;59(3):613–6.

17. Su LM, Goldstein M, Schlegel PN. The effect of varicocelectomy on serum testosterone levels in infertile men with varicoceles. J Urol 1995;154:1752–5.

18. Cayan S, Kadioglu A, Orhan I, et al. The effect of microsurgical varicocelectomy on serum follicle stimulating hormone, testosterone and free testosterone levels in infertile men with varicocele. BJU Int 1999;84(9):1046–9.

19. Gat Y, Gornish M, Belenky A, et al. Elevation of serum testosterone and free testosterone after embolization of the internal spermatic vein for the treatment of varicocele in infertile men. Hum Reprod 2004;19(10):2303–6.

20. Pierik FH, Abdesselam SA, Vreeburg JT, et al. Increased serum inhibin B levels after varicocele treatment. Clin Endocrinol (Oxf) 2001;54(6):775–80.

21. Resorlu B, Kara C, Sahin E, et al. The significance of age on success of surgery for patients with varicocele. Int Urol Nephrol 2010;42(2):351–6.

22. Rodriguez Peña M, Alescio L, Russell A, et al. Predictors of improved seminal parameters and fertility after varicocele repair in young adults. Andrologia 2009;41(5):277–81.

23. Al-Ali B, Shamloul R, Pichler M, et al. Clinical and laboratory profiles of a large cohort of patients with different grades of varicocele. Cent European J Urol 2013;66(1):71–4.

24. Hsiao W, Rosoff JS, Pale JR, et al. Older age is associated with similar improvements in semen parameters and testosterone after subinguinal microsurgical varicocelectomy. J Urol 2011;185(2):620–5.

25. Di Bisceglie C, Bertagna A, Baldi M, et al. Varicocele sclerotherapy improves serum inhibin B levels and seminal parameters. Int J Androl 2007;30(6):531–6.

26. Tanrikut C, Goldstein M, Rosoff JS, et al. Varicocele as a risk factor for androgen deficiency and effect of repair. BJU Int 2011;108(9):1480–4.

27. Sathya Srini V, Belur Veerachari S. Does varicocelectomy improve gonadal function in men with hypogonadism and infertility? Analysis of a prospective study. Int J Endocrinol 2011;2011:916380.

28. Abdel-Meguid TA, Farsi HM, Al-Sayyad A, et al. Effects of varicocele on serum testosterone and changes of testosterone after varicocelectomy: a prospective controlled study. Urology 2014;84(5):1081–7.

29. Ahmed A, Abdel-Aziz A, Maarouf A, et al. The impact of varicocelectomy on premature ejaculation in varicocele patients. Andrologia 2015;47(3):276–81.

30. Shabana W, Teleb M, Dawod T, et al. Predictors of improvement in semen parameters after varicocelectomy for male subfertility: a prospective study. Can Urol Assoc J 2015;9(9–10):E579–82.

31. Zohdy W, Ghazi S, Arafa M. Impact of varicocelectomy on gonadal and erectile functions in men with hypogonadism and infertility. J Sex Med 2011;8(3):885–93.

32. Hudson RW, Perez-Marrero RA, Crawford VA, et al. Hormonal parameters of men with varicoceles before and after varicocelectomy. Fertil Steril 1985;43(6):905–10.

33. Sweeney TE, Rozum JS, Gore RW. Alteration of testicular microvascular pressures during venous pressure elevation. Am J Physiol Heart Circ Physiol 1995;269(1):H37–45. Available at: http://ajpheart.physiology.org/content/269/1/H37.short.

34. Shiraishi K, Takihara H, Matsuyama H. Elevated scrotal temperature, but not varicocele grade, reflects testicular oxidative stress-mediated apoptosis. World J Urol 2010;28:359–64.

35. Diemer T, Allen JA, Hales KH, et al. Reactive oxygen disrupts mitochondria in MA-10 tumor Leydig cells and inhibits steroidogenic acute regulatory (StAR) protein and steroidogenesis. Endocrinology 2003;144(7):2882–91.

36. Stocco DM, Wells J, Clark BJ. The effects of hydrogen peroxide on steroidogenesis in mouse Leydig tumor cells. Endocrinology 1993;133(6):2827–32.

37. Hudson RW, McKay DE. The gonadotropin response of men with varicoceles to gonadotropin-releasing hormone. Fertil Steril 1980;33(4):427–32.

38. Ando S, Giacchetto C, Beraldi E, et al. Progesterone, 17-OH-progesterone, androstenedione and testosterone plasma levels in spermatic venous blood of normal men and varicocele patients. Horm Metab Res 1985;17(2):99–103.

39. Gomes WR, Butler WR, Johnson AD. Effect of elevated ambient temperature on testis and blood levels and in vitro biosynthesis of testosterone in the ram. J Anim Sci 1971;33(4):804–7.

40. Goldstein M, Eid JF. Elevation of intratesticular and scrotal skin surface temperature in men with varicocele. J Urol 1989;142(3):743–5.

41. Scholler R, Nahoul K, Castanier M, et al. Testicular secretion of conjugated and unconjugated steroids in normal adults and in patients with varicocele. Baseline levels and time-course response to hCG administration. J Steroid Biochem 1984; 20(1):203–15.

42. Sirvent JJ, Bernat R, Navarro MA, et al. Leydig cell in idiopathic varicocele. Eur Urol 1990;17(3):257–61.

43. Francavilla S, Bruno B, Martini M, et al. Quantitative evaluation of Leydig cells in testicular biopsies of men with varicocele. Arch Androl 1986;16(2): 111–7.

44. Weiss DB, Rodriguez-Rigau L, Smith KD, et al. Quantitation of Leydig cells in testicular biopsies of oligospermic men with varicocele. Fertil Steril 1978;30:305–12.

45. Gat Y, Bachar GN, Zukerman Z, et al. Varicocele: a bilateral disease. Fertil Steril 2004;81(2):424–9.

46. Page ST. Physiologic role and regulation of intratesticular sex steroids. Curr Opin Endocrinol Diabetes Obes 2011;18(3):217–23.

47. Gu Y, Liang X, Wu W, et al. Multicenter contraceptive efficacy trial of injectable testosterone undecanoate in Chinese men. J Clin Endocrinol Metab 2009;94(6): 1910–5.

48. Hendin BN, Kolettis PN, Sharma RK, et al. Varicocele is associated with elevated spermatozoal reactive oxygen species production and diminished seminal plasma antioxidant capacity. J Urol 1999; 161(6):1831–4.

49. Mostafa T, Anis TH, El-Nashar A, et al. Varicocelectomy reduces reactive oxygen species levels and increases antioxidant activity of seminal plasma from infertile men with varicocele. Int J Androl 2001; 24(5):261–5.

50. Saleh RA, Agarwal A, Sharma RK, et al. Evaluation of nuclear DNA damage in spermatozoa from infertile men with varicocele. Fertil Steril 2003;80(6): 1431–6.

51. Hurtado de Catalfo GE, Ranieri-Casilla A, Marra FA, et al. Oxidative stress biomarkers and hormonal profile in human patients undergoing varicocelectomy. Int J Androl 2007;30(6):519–30.

52. Rajfer J, Turner TT, Rivera F, et al. Inhibition of testicular testosterone biosynthesis following experimental varicocele in rats. Biol Reprod 1987;36(4): 933–7.

53. Zheng Y, Zhang X, Zhou J, et al. Effects on the ipsilateral testis during progression of experimental varicocele in rat. Med Sci Monit 2008;14(6):BR122–6.

54. Ozturk MI, Koca O, Keles MO, et al. The impact of unilateral experimental rat varicocele model on testicular histopathology, Leydig cell counts, and intratesticular testosterone levels of both testes. Urol J 2013;10(3):973–80.

55. Luo D-Y, Yang G, Liu J-J, et al. Effects of varicocele on testosterone, apoptosis and expression of StAR mRNA in rat Leydig cells. Asian J Androl 2011; 13(2):287–91.

56. Zheng Y-Q, Zhang X-B, Zhou J-Q, et al. The effects of artery-ligating and artery-preserving varicocelectomy on the ipsilateral testes in rats. Urology 2008; 72(5):1179–84.

57. Shafik A, Wali MA, Abdel Azis YE, et al. Experimental model of varicocele. Eur Urol 1989;16(4): 298–303.

58. Ghosh PK, York JP. Changes in testicular testosterone and acid and alkaline phosphatase activity in testis and accessory sex organs after induction of varicocele in noble rats. J Surg Res 1994;56(3): 271–6.

59. Sweeney TE, Rozum JS, Desjardins C, et al. Microvascular pressure distribution in the hamster testis. Am J Physiol 1991;260(5 Pt 2):H1581–9.

60. Zalata AA, Mokhtar N, Badawy AE, et al. Androgen receptor expression relationship with semen variables in infertile men with varicocele. J Urol 2013; 189(6):2243–7.

61. Soares TS, Fernandes SA, Lima ML, et al. Experimental varicocoele in rats affects mechanisms that control expression and function of the androgen receptor. Andrology 2013;1(5):670–81.

62. Younes AK. Improvement of sexual activity, pregnancy rate, and low plasma testosterone after bilateral varicocelectomy in impotence and male infertility patients. Arch Androl 2003;49(3):219–28.

63. Lotti F, Corona G, Mancini M, et al. The association between varicocele, premature ejaculation and prostatitis symptoms: possible mechanisms. J Sex Med 2009;6(10):2878–87.

64. Smith JF, Walsh TJ, Shindel AW, et al. Sexual, marital, and social impact of a man's perceived infertility diagnosis. J Sex Med 2009;6(9):2505–15.

65. Wischmann TH. Sexual disorders in infertile couples. J Sex Med 2010;7(5):1868–76.

66. Keller JJ, Chen Y-K, Lin H-C. Varicocele is associated with erectile dysfunction: a population-based case-control study. J Sex Med 2012;9(7): 1745–52.

67. Liu X, Zhang H, Ruan X, et al. Macroscopic and microsurgical varicocelectomy: what's the intraoperative difference? World J Urol 2013;31(3): 603–8.

68. Hsiao W, Rosoff JS, Pale JR, et al. Varicocelectomy is associated with increases in serum testosterone independent of clinical grade. Urology 2013;81(6): 1213–7.

69. Ozden C, Ozdal OL, Bulut S, et al. Effect of varicocelectomy on serum inhibin B levels in infertile patients with varicocele. Scand J Urol Nephrol 2008; 42(5):441–3.

70. Fujisawa M, Dobashi M, Yamasaki T, et al. Significance of serum inhibin B concentration for evaluating improvement in spermatogenesis after varicocelectomy. Hum Reprod 2001;16(9):1945–9.

Testosterone Deficiency and Sleep Apnea

Omar Burschtin, MD[a], Jing Wang, MD[b],*

KEYWORDS

- Obstructive sleep apnea • Testosterone deficiency • Sexual dysfunction
- Continuous positive airway pressure

KEY POINTS

- Obstructive sleep apnea (OSA) is associated with altered pituitary–gonadal function.
- Serum testosterone (T) has been shown to be lower in men with OSA.
- T supplementation may alter ventilatory responses and reduce sensitivity to hypercapnea.
- OSA may be a risk factor for erectile and sexual dysfunction in men.
- Treatment of OSA may help improve hypogonadism and sexual function.

INTRODUCTION

Obstructive sleep apnea (OSA) is a common condition among middle-aged men, affecting approximately 25% of men over the age of 40 (apnea hypopnea index [AHI] >5).[1] When looking at more subtle divisions of OSA severity, 18% of men in this age group still fall within the mild category, at AHI greater than 10, and 11% have at least moderate disease, with AHI greater than 15. This disorder is characterized by repetitive collapse of the airway during sleep, resulting in oxygen desaturation and sleep fragmentation. Observational studies have shown that OSA is a risk factor for cardiovascular morbidity, including hypertension, coronary heart disease, and stroke.[2–4] Sleep-disordered breathing has also been associated with altered pituitary–gonadal function. This article discusses the relationship between OSA and testosterone (T) deficiency.

Studies evaluating the relationship between T and sleep date back to the 1970s.[5–7] One of the earlier studies measured T and luteinizing hormone (LH) every 20 minutes for 24 hours in 9 pubertal boys and 3 sexually mature young men, and found that T levels fluctuated over the course of the day, with pubertal boys showing an increase in LH and T secretion during sleep. When the sleep–wake cycle was reversed, this pattern held true. However, this effect was not seen in sexually mature men. Another study evaluated T levels in men aged 22 to 32 years after night sleep and daytime sleep, and found an increase in T levels during any period of sleep and a decrease during waking hours, independent of circadian timing.[8] These studies suggest that LH-T augmentation during sleep is an important component of normal male physiology.

LOW TESTOSTERONE AND SLEEP APNEA: ROLES OF AGE, BODY MASS INDEX, AND SEVERITY OF SLEEP APNEA

Serum T has been shown to be lower in men with OSA.[9] Multiple studies describe a negative correlation between polysomnographic parameters—AHI, oxygen desaturation index (ODI), and nadir oxygen saturation - and testosterone levels.[10,11] A study by Luboshitzky and colleagues, measuring LH and T between 7 p.m. and 7 a.m. in obese men with OSA, obese men without OSA, and lean healthy men, found LH and T to be significantly lower in obese men with OSA compared with lean controls. Furthermore, both men with

[a] Mount Sinai School of Medicine, Division of Pulmonary, Critical Care and Sleep Medicine, 11 East 26th Street, 13th Floor, New York, NY 10010, USA; [b] NYU School of Medicine, Division of Pulmonary, Critical Care, and Sleep Medicine, 462 First Avenue Room 7N24, New York, NY 10016, USA
* Corresponding author.
E-mail address: jing.wang@nyumc.org

Urol Clin N Am 43 (2016) 233–237
http://dx.doi.org/10.1016/j.ucl.2016.01.012
0094-0143/16/$ – see front matter © 2016 Elsevier Inc. All rights reserved.

OSA and middle-aged controls had less pulsatile T release and reduced LH pulse amplitude, suggesting that, beyond the presence of OSA, obesity and age also play a role in androgen secretion.[12]

LOW TESTOSTERONE AND SLEEP APNEA: ROLE OF FATIGUE

Fatigue is a common reported symptom in OSA, even in the absence of daytime sleepiness.[13] Bercea and colleagues investigated the relationship between fatigue, OSA, and T levels in 2 groups consisting of OSA patients and age- and body mass index (BMI)-matched controls without OSA. In addition to lower serum testosterone, severe OSA patients also had more general fatigue, physical fatigue, mental fatigue, and reduced activity. In multivariate analyses, T level was the only independent predictor of physical fatigue and reduced activity in the OSA group. Of note, nadir oxygen saturation was not a significant predictor of fatigue. This study suggests that T deficiency in men with OSA has multiple health consequences, and fatigue may be an important factor affecting quality of life in this cohort.[14]

EFFECT OF TESTOSTERONE SUPPLEMENTATION ON OBSTRUCTIVE SLEEP APNEA

Untreated OSA has been considered a contraindication to T therapy, as it is believed that T replacement therapy (TRT) can worsen sleep apnea. Several studies have investigated the role of T administration in OSA. A case study by Cistulli and colleagues[15] reported that administration of high-dose T to a 13-year-old boy exacerbated OSA due to neuromuscular collapse of upper airway during sleep. Schneider and colleagues[16] found an increase in the number of apneas and hypopneas and a corresponding rise in AHI following androgen administration to hypogonadal males. These changes were noted without significant changes in upper airway dimensions or alterations in sleep stage distribution.

Matsumoto and colleagues[17] evaluated the effect of 6 weeks of biweekly 200 mg intramuscular T enanthate injections on hypoxic and hypercapnic ventilatory drive (ie, increase in ventilation induced by hypoxia or hypercapnea) in 5 hypogonadal men. Hypoxic ventilatory drive decreased significantly, while hypercapnic ventilatory drive did not. OSA developed in 1 subject and worsened in another. Both these patients showed a decrease in oxygen saturation, development of cardiac dysrhythmias during sleep, and an increase in hematocrit. On retrospective review of another group of elderly hypogonadal men with 2-year follow-up, a significant increase in hematocrit was seen, with 24% of men developing polycythemia (hematocrit [Hct] >52%) requiring phlebotomy or temporary cessation of testosterone therapy. No significant change in sleep-disordered breathing was reported, however.[18]

In a larger, randomized, placebo-controlled, cross-over trial of short-term high-dose T therapy, otherwise healthy participants with baseline T levels less than 450 ng/dL were given weekly injections of T (500 mg, 250 mg, 250 mg) and underwent polysomnographic testing and assessment of anthropometrics and airway bioimpedance. T treatment reduced rapid eye movement (REM) and non-REM (NREM) sleep by approximately 1 hour, although the proportion of time spent in each stage did not change significantly. RDI was increased by approximately 7 events per hour, and duration of hypoxemia was prolonged by T treatment. Interestingly, no significant change was seen in upper airway caliber, measured by awake acoustic reflectometry, or in neck and abdominal circumference. Rather, there was a reduction in serum leptin levels and adiposity, pointing to less pharyngeal fat deposition as a mechanism for the change in respiratory parameters.[19]

In a subsequent study, the same group studied obese adult men with OSA randomized to 3 intramuscular injections of T or placebo at 0, 6, and 12 weeks, and measured ventilatory chemoreflexes, including response to hypercapnea. They found a significant correlation between the hyperoxic carbon dioxide ventilatory recruitment threshold and increase in serum testosterone level at 6 weeks, indicating a dampened response to hypercapnea, along with a corresponding increase in time spent below oxygen saturation of 90% in sleep. A similar trend was seen for the ventilatory response in hypoxic conditions. This effect, however, did not persist on later measurements at week 18. The mechanism for this time-dependent difference in response remains to be better elucidated, although the findings suggest perhaps an effect of T on central chemoreceptors.[20]

MEN WITH OBSTRUCTIVE SLEEP APNEA AND SEXUAL DYSFUNCTION

There is growing evidence for an association between OSA and sexual dysfunction. Early observational data from Guilleminault and colleagues[21] indicated a high prevalence (48%) of erectile dysfunction (ED) in men with severe OSA. Margel and colleagues[22] also found a significant correlation between presence of ED and severe OSA, although the relationship was weaker in patients with mild or moderate disease. Composite results from a recent meta-analysis reported a relative risk of 1.82 for ED in men with OSA.[23]

EFFECT OF OBSTRUCTIVE SLEEP APNEA TREATMENT ON TESTOSTERONE LEVEL

The data investigating whether treating OSA results in an increase in T levels are mixed. One case series of 12 men with moderate-to-severe OSA who underwent uvulopalatopharyngoplasty (UPPP) showed small increases in T levels and improvement in self-reported sexual function 3 months after surgery without significant changes in prolactin, LH, or follicle-stimulating hormone (FSH) levels.[24] In another longitudinal study of 43 patients with severe OSA who were treated with nasal continuous positive airway pressure (CPAP), a significant increase in total T and sex hormone binding globulin (SHBG) was seen after 3 months of therapy, again suggesting a reversible component to the neuroendocrine dysfunction seen with OSA.[25] A randomized trial of 101 men with OSA who were given either therapeutic or sham CPAP showed that T and SHBG were negatively correlated to OSA severity at baseline. CPAP treatment did not increase T levels, but did result in SHBG elevation, along with increases in aldosterone and insulin-like growth factor 1 (IGF-1). The main drawback of this study was the short follow-up time of only 1 month.[25]

There are more positive data pointing to an improvement in sexual dysfunction with OSA treatment, independent of T levels. A study of 98 men with OSA found that those with ED had generally higher AHIs, lower oxygen saturation during sleep, and higher Epworth Sleepiness Scale and Beck Depression Inventory scores. These differences were eliminated with nasal CPAP treatment, and ED resolved in 75% of patients.[26] Another study that included over 200 patients also reported lower baseline T levels and International Index of Erectile Dysfunction-5 (IIEF-5) scores in men with severe OSA.[27] There were no significant differences in other hormones, including prolactin, LH, FSH, and estradiol. Three months of treatment with CPAP improved the IIEF-5 scores significantly, but did not result in changes in sexual hormone levels. Interestingly, a trial by Hoekema and colleagues[28] found no significant change in subjective measures of sexual function in a group of men with varying degrees of OSA when treated with either CPAP or an oral appliance.

In some of these patients with sexual dysfunction, there may be a benefit for using TRT. A pilot study evaluated TRT, PDE-5 inhibitor use, and CPAP in men with OSA and ED confirmed by nocturnal penile tumescence examination.[29] In the patients with normal T levels at baseline, use of a PDE-5 inhibitor alone was sufficient to correct ED (success rate >75%) after 6 months of therapy. However, in hypogonadal men, those treated with a combination of TRT, PDE-5 inhibitor, and CPAP did best, with normal erectile function after 3 months, compared with those who received PDE-5 inhibitor alone (only 42% showed improvement after 3 months). This suggests a positive additive benefit of TRT to PDE-5 inhibitors in hypogonadal men with OSA who receive CPAP therapy. It remains unclear whether TRT without CPAP would achieve a similar benefit. Larger, controlled studies are still needed.

OBSTRUCTIVE SLEEP APNEA AND POLYCYTHEMIA

Conditions of chronic hypoxemia, such as advanced lung disease and high altitude exposure, are known causes of polycythemia and cor pulmonale. OSA is characterized by repetitive periods of intermittent hypoxia, which has been proposed to be another risk factor for secondary polycythemia or erythrocytosis. Carlson and colleagues[30] described an increased prevalence of sleep-disordered breathing among patients with unexplained polycythemia in the absence of a difference in erythropoietin levels. In a larger study, Hoffstein and colleagues found a weak association between sleep apnea and increased Hct levels. Patients with more severe sleep apnea and longer periods of low nocturnal oxygen saturation (below 85%) appeared to have marginally higher Hct, although none reached polycythemic levels of Hct greater than 55%.[31] A subsequent investigation by Choi and colleagues found a significant correlation between Hct and respiratory disturbance index (RDI), another marker of OSA severity, mean oxygen saturation, and sleep time below oxygen saturation of 90%. Moreover, patients with severe OSA (RDI >30) had higher Hct than patients with mild-to-moderate disease (Hct 43.5% vs 41.2%), even after adjusting for gender, ethnicity, BMI, blood pressure, and catecholamine levels. Again, however, no clinically significant polycythemia was detected, suggesting that Hct is less useful as a screening tool for OSA.[32]

Up to 20% to 30% of patients with OSA also have concurrent obesity hypoventilation, characterized by chronic hypercapnea and sustained nocturnal hypoxemia.[33,34] Similar to patients with chronic obstructive pulmonary disease (COPD), secondary erythrocytosis has been described in patients with chronic alveolar hypoventilation, usually associated with states of prolonged hypoxemia.[35,36] It is possible that hypoxia-induced vascular growth factors play a role in this up-regulation of erythrocytes.[37] Therefore, evaluation for underlying causes of hypoventilation, in addition to OSA, is often recommended as part of the work-up for secondary polycythemia.[38] Importantly, this relationship should be kept in mind when considering the patient with OSA and hypogonadism who is considering T replacement, as T replacement is known to exacerbate polycythemia in some patients.

Interestingly, a few small studies have described a decrease in hematocrit levels with OSA treatment.[39] Krieger and colleagues measured Hct and red cell count before and after a single night of nasal CPAP therapy in a group of 8 patients with sleep apnea and found a small reduction in both parameters post-therapy (Hct 45.6% vs 43%). In a follow-up study, the same group tracked patients with unequivocal OSA (AHI >30/h) over the course of 1 year before and after CPAP therapy. They again found a decrease in Hct following just 1 night of CPAP therapy, with rebound effects seen off positive airway pressure. Hct remained in the range of the initial post-treatment baseline value on long-term follow-up (42.4% vs 42.9%). The mechanism of these effects remains unclear, with several hypotheses proposed, including fluid shifts and changes in red cell volume.[40,41]

SUMMARY

The relationships between T and OSA are complex and not yet completely understood. Available evidence points to reduced T levels in men with OSA, along with higher incidence of fatigue and sexual dysfunction. Some of the proposed mechanisms explaining this effect are alteration of sleep architecture, periods of low oxygen saturation in sleep, and changes in control hormone levels. There is concern that TRT, when given in high doses or alone without adequate treatment of OSA, may further compromise respiratory and polysomnographic parameters, with or without significant changes in airway dynamics. On the other hand, treatment of OSA may help improve sexual function, especially in men with severe disease. Additional systematic investigation of these clinically important questions is needed.

REFERENCES

1. Young T, Palta M, Dempsey J, et al. The occurrence of sleep-disordered breathing among middle-aged adults. N Engl J Med 1993;328:1230–5.

2. Nieto FJ, Young TB, Lind BK, et al. Association of sleep-disordered breathing, sleep apnea, and hypertension in a large community-based study: sleep heart health study. JAMA 2000;283:1829–36 [Erratum appears in JAMA 2002;288:1985].

3. Gottlieb DJ, Yenokyan G, Newman AB, et al. Prospective study of obstructive sleep apnea and incident coronary heart disease and heart failure: the sleep heart health study. Circulation 2010;122: 352–60.

4. Redline S, Yenokyan G, Gottlieb DJ, et al. Obstructive sleep apnea–hypopnea and incident stroke: the sleep heart health study. Am J Respir Crit Care Med 2010;182:269–77.

5. Boyar RM, Rosenfeld RS, Kapen S, et al. Human puberty. simultaneous augmented secretion of luteinizing hormone and testosterone during sleep. J Clin Invest 1974;54(3):609–18.

6. Camargo CA. Obstructive sleep apnea and testosterone. N Engl J Med 1983;309(5):314–5.

7. Evans JI, MacLean AW, Ismail AA, et al. Concentrations of plasma testosterone in normal men during sleep. Nature 1971;229(5282):261–2.

8. Axelsson J, Ingre M, Akerstedt T, et al. Effects of acutely displaced sleep on testosterone. J Clin Endocrinol Metab 2005;90(8):4530–5.

9. Canguven O, Salepci B, Albayrak S, et al. Is there a correlation between testosterone levels and the severity of the disease in male patients with obstructive sleep apnea? Arch Ital Urol Androl 2010;82(4): 143–7.

10. Gambineri A, Pelusi C, Pasquali R. Testosterone levels in obese male patients with obstructive sleep apnea syndrome: relation to oxygen desaturation, body weight, fat distribution and the metabolic parameters. J Endocrinol Invest 2003;26(6):493–8.

11. Hammoud AO, Walker JM, Gibson M, et al. Sleep apnea, reproductive hormones and quality of sexual life in severely obese men. Obesity (Silver Spring) 2011;19(6):1118–23.

12. Luboshitzky R, Lavie L, Shen-Orr Z, et al. Altered luteinizing hormone and testosterone secretion in middle-aged obese men with obstructive sleep apnea. Obes Res 2005;13(4):780–6.

13. Chervin R. Sleepiness, fatigue, tiredness, and lack of energy in obstructive sleep apnea. Chest 2000; 118(2):372–9.

14. Bercea RM, Mihaescu T, Cojocaru C, et al. Fatigue and serum testosterone in obstructive sleep apnea patients. Clin Respir J 2015;9(3):342–9.

15. Cistulli PA, Grunstein RR, Sullivan CE. Effect of testosterone administration on upper airway collapsibility during sleep. Am J Respir Crit Care Med 1994; 149(2 Pt 1):530–2.

16. Schneider BK, Pickett CK, Zwillich CW, et al. Influence of testosterone on breathing during sleep. J Appl Physiol (1985) 1986;61(2):618–23.

17. Matsumoto AM, Sandblom RE, Schoene RB, et al. Testosterone replacement in hypogonadal men: effects on obstructive sleep apnoea, respiratory drives, and sleep. Clin Endocrinol (Oxf) 1985; 22(6):713–21.

18. Hajjar RR, Kaiser FE, Morley JE. Outcomes of long-term testosterone replacement in older hypogonadal males: a retrospective analysis. J Clin Endocrinol Metab 1997;82(11):3793–6.

19. Liu PY, Yee B, Wishart SM, et al. The short-term effects of high-dose testosterone on sleep, breathing, and function in older men. J Clin Endocrinol Metab 2003;88(8):3605–13.

20. Killick R, Wang D, Hoyos CM, et al. The effects of testosterone on ventilatory responses in men with obstructive sleep apnea: a randomised, placebo-controlled trial. J Sleep Res 2013;22(3):331–6.

21. Guilleminault C, Simmons FB, Motta J, et al. Obstructive sleep apnea syndrome and tracheostomy. Long-term follow-up experience. Arch Intern Med 1981;141:985–8.

22. Margel D, Cohen M, Livne PM, et al. Severe, but not mild, obstructive sleep apnea syndrome is associated with erectile dysfunction. Urology 2004;63: 545–9.

23. Liu L, Kang R, Zhao S, et al. Sexual dysfunction in patients with obstructive sleep apnea: a systematic review and meta-analysis. J Sex Med 2015;12(10): 1992–2003.

24. Santamaria JD, Prior JC, Fleetham JA. Reversible reproductive dysfunction in men with obstructive sleep apnoea. Clin Endocrinol (Oxf) 1988;28(5): 461–70.

25. Grunstein RR, Handelsman DJ, Lawrence SJ, et al. Neuroendocrine dysfunction in sleep apnea: reversal by continuous positive airways pressure therapy. J Clin Endocrinol Metab 1989;68(2):352–8.

26. Goncalves MA, Guilleminault C, Ramos E, et al. Erectile dysfunction, obstructive sleep apnea syndrome and nasal CPAP treatment. Sleep Med 2005;6(4):333–9.

27. Zhang XB, Lin QC, Zeng HQ, et al. Erectile dysfunction and sexual hormone levels in men with obstructive sleep apnea: efficacy of continuous positive airway pressure. Arch Sex Behav 2015;45(1):235–40.

28. Hoekema A, Stel AL, Stegenga B, et al. Sexual function and obstructive sleep apnea-hypopnea: a randomized clinical trial evaluating the effects of oral-appliance and continuous positive airway pressure therapy. J Sex Med 2007;4:1153–62.

29. Zhuravlev VN, Frank MA, Gomzhin AI. Sexual functions of men with obstructive sleep apnoea syndrome and hypogonadism may improve upon testosterone administration: a pilot study. Andrologia 2009;41(3):193–5.

30. Carlson JT, Hedner J, Fagerberg B, et al. Secondary polycythaemia associated with nocturnal apnoea–a relationship not mediated by erythropoietin? J Intern Med 1992;231(4):381–7.

31. Hoffstein V, Herridge M, Mateika S, et al. Hematocrit levels in sleep apnea. Chest 1994;106(3):787–91.

32. Choi JB, Loredo JS, Norman D, et al. Does obstructive sleep apnea increase hematocrit? Sleep Breath 2006;10:155–6.

33. Dabal L, BaHamman AS. Obesity hypoventilation syndrome. Ann Thorac Med 2009;4(2):41–9.

34. Mokhlesi B, Tulaimat A, Faibussowitsch I, et al. Obesity hypoventilation syndrome: prevalence and predictors in patients with obstructive sleep apnea. Sleep Breath 2007;11(2):117–24.

35. Lawrence T. Idiopathic hypoventilation, polycythemia, and cor pulmonale. Am Rev Respir Dis 1959;80(4):575–81.

36. Kent BD, Mitchell PD, McNicholas WT. Hypoxemia in patients with COPD: cause, effects, and disease progression. Int J Chron Obstruct Pulmon Dis 2011;6:199–208.

37. Semenza GL. Regulation of oxygen homeostasis by hypoxia-inducible factor 1. Physiology 2009;24: 97–106.

38. Lee G, Arcasoy MO. The clinical and laboratory evaluation of the patient with erythrocytosis. Eur J Intern Med 2015;26(5):297–302.

39. Krieger J, Sforza E, Delanoe C, et al. Decrease in hematocrit with continuous positive airway pressure treatment in obstructive sleep apnea patients. Eur Respir J 1992;5:228–33.

40. Saarelainen S, Hasan J, Seppala E. Effect of nasal CPAP treatment on plasma volume, aldosterone and 24-h blood pressure in obstructive sleep apnea. J Sleep Res 1996;5:181–5.

41. Krieger J, Follenius M, Sforza E, et al. Effects of treatment with nasal continuous positive airway pressure on atrial natriuretic peptide and arginine vasopressin release during sleep in obstructive sleep apnea. Clin Sci 1991;80:443–9.

Obesity and Hypogonadism

Steven Lamm, MD*, Aaron Chidakel, MD, Rohan Bansal, BA

KEYWORDS

• Obesity • Hypogonadism • Testosterone • Diabetes

KEY POINTS

- The relationship between obesity and hypogonadism is bidirectional and there are numerous causative and correlative factors on both sides of the equation.
- Obesity is growing in prevalence in epidemic proportions. Likewise, we are beginning to see the rapid increase in the incidence of male hypogonadism.
- It is only recently that we are learning the ways in which these 2 conditions exacerbate each other.
- We are only beginning to understand how by treating one of these conditions, we can help to treat the other, as well.

INTRODUCTION

It will not be surprising to most people how ubiquitous obesity is today, both in America and throughout the world. Nor should it be surprising how frequently male hypogonadism is diagnosed in recent years. What is of great interest, however, are the mechanisms by which these 2 increasingly prevalent conditions may interact with and exacerbate each other. It is also important to understand how by treating one of these conditions, we may be able to help alleviate the effects of the other as well.

In recent times, obesity has become a global epidemic: the prevalence of obesity has rapidly increased, and obesity-related comorbidities have surged over the past few decades. It is estimated that more than one-third (34.9% or 78.6 million) of U.S. adults are obese and more than two-thirds of U.S adults are overweight.[1] Obesity is known to lead to other comorbidities, such as hypertension, dyslipidemia, type 2 diabetes mellitus, coronary heart disease, stroke, gallbladder disease, osteoarthritis, sleep apnea, respiratory problems, as well as chronic liver disorders like nonalcoholic fatty liver disease and its most severe subset, nonalcoholic steatohepatitis.[2–4]

It is also important to note that, although much work remains with regard to treatment of obesity, this field has rapidly developed over the past decade. It is no longer appropriate to simply surrender when a patient is unable to lose weight through diet and exercise alone and tell him that we can no longer help him. The specifics of the pharmacologic approaches to treatment of obesity are beyond the scope of this article and may be found in detailed form elsewhere.[5]

In addition to these sequelae, hypogonadism is an important comorbidity of obesity that is often overlooked. Hypogonadism, defined as the presence of low testosterone level measured on at least 2 occasions along with signs or symptoms that are owing to low testosterone, has been shown to be strongly correlated with obesity.[5] In fact, it has been reported that obesity is probably the single most common cause of testosterone deficiency in the developed world, with approximately 52.4% of all obese men having testosterone levels below 300 ng/dL.[6] Likewise, weight loss, as a result of diet, exercise, or bariatric

Department of Medicine, NYU Langone Preston Robert Tisch Center for Men's Health, 555 Madison Avenue, 2nd Floor, New York, NY 10022, USA
* Corresponding author.
E-mail address: Steven.Lamm@nyumc.org

Urol Clin N Am 43 (2016) 239–245
http://dx.doi.org/10.1016/j.ucl.2016.01.005
0094-0143/16/$ – see front matter © 2016 Elsevier Inc. All rights reserved.

surgery, can significantly increase testosterone levels in men.[7] In addition to promoting obesity, hypogonadism has been implicated with a number of other sequelae as well, including sexual dysfunction, osteoporosis, depression, dyslipidemia, and the metabolic syndrome.[8]

Interestingly, the relationship between obesity and hypogonadism seems to be bidirectional, because there is an increase in deposition of abdominal adipose tissue in hypogonadal subjects.[9] Furthermore, there is evidence to suggest that testosterone replacement therapy may improve body fat mass, waist circumference, and muscle mass, and may thereby be a potential treatment modality for obesity.[10,11]

Clearly the relationship between hypogonadism and obesity is complicated and questions remain surrounding the degree of correlation and causality between the 2 conditions. What is known is that these 2 conditions have been discovered to coexist with frequency and treatment of one of these conditions may confer potential benefits on the other. There are numerous speculations as to the physiology behind these mechanisms.

The first step to understanding the complex relationship between obesity and hypogonadism is to take a closer look at the underlying driver of obesity itself, namely, adipose tissue. Whereas adipose tissue, or fat, was once considered to simply be a reservoir for storage of high-energy fuels, it is now understood to be a complex, essential, and highly active metabolic and endocrine organ.[12]

ADIPOSE TISSUE AS AN ORGAN

The traditional view of adipose tissue storage has changed over the past 20 years from that of a pure reservoir for energy to what we now recognize as a complex and highly active endocrine and metabolic organ, responding to incoming signals from both the central nervous system and various glands by expressing and secreting essential active proteins. It is also now well-known that adipose tissue is a major site for the metabolism of sex steroids and glucocorticoids. To better understand this relationship, we will analyze the function of adipose tissue with respect to the hormones it regulates and produces, and the different types of adipose tissue that exist.

As an endocrine and metabolic organ, adipose tissue expresses and secretes active metabolic factors, such as leptin, tumor necrosis factor (TNF)-alpha, interleukin (IL)-6 and adiponectin.[13] Leptin, the "satiety hormone," is a hormone made by adipocytes that helps to regulate energy balance by inhibiting hunger.[14] Although the majority of leptin's effects are mediated via hypothalamic

pathways, some are mediated directly by peripheral tissues, including muscle cells and pancreatic beta cells. It is known that, with caloric restriction and weight loss, leptin levels decrease quickly, leading to an increase of appetite and lower basal level of energy expenditure. This response is preserved in morbidly obese humans who are leptin deficient, and returns to normal if low-dose leptin replacement is given. In turn, obesity is typically associated with increased levels of leptin, which do not decrease after administration of exogenous leptin, suggesting that these individuals are leptin resistant.[15]

TNF-alpha is also expressed in adipose tissue, and is implicated in causing obesity and insulin resistance. Plasma levels of TNF-alpha have been positively correlated with obesity in some studies.[16] As of late, attention has focused on the adipose tissue production TNF-alpha in metabolic syndrome and type 2 diabetes mellitus, as the levels are elevated, creating a proinflammatory state associated with insulin resistance and endothelial dysfunction.[17] Furthermore, higher levels of TNF-alpha (as well as other proinflammatory cytokines) may influence the secretion of pituitary gonadotropins.[18]

Likewise, IL-6 is another protein that is expressed by adipose tissue and is associated with obesity and insulin resistance.[13] In fact, it has been reported that a sedentary lifestyle may be accompanied by the infiltration of immune cells with proinflammatory characteristics in adipose tissue, causing an increased release of cytokines such as IL-6 and generating a low-grade inflammatory state. This in turn, may lead to such conditions as insulin resistance, and this may improve with reduction of fat mass.[19]

Adiponectin, on the other hand, is a hormone derived from adipose tissue that seems to convey protection from cardiovascular disease and increased insulin sensitivity; it also has a beneficial effect on postprandial glucose and lipid metabolism.[20] In contrast with the majority of the other adipokines that have been identified, plasma levels of adiponectin are decreased significantly in obese patients, and are negatively correlated with body mass index.[21]

Over the years, we have also come to understand that the function of adipose tissue is largely determined by its location. Visceral adipose tissue secretes its endocrine hormones directly into the portal system, whereas subcutaneous tissue secretes into systemic circulation. Hence, visceral adiposity has a greater effect on hepatic metabolic function. Expression of IL-6 is higher in visceral adipose tissue, whereas expression of leptin is higher in subcutaneous tissue. Finally, these different types of tissue respond differently to afferent signals, largely because visceral tissue has higher levels of glucocorticoid and androgen receptors. Most interesting, however, is that visceral fat is associated with increased metabolic risk and mortality, whereas subcutaneous fat expansion actually improves insulin sensitivity, and reduces the risk of type 2 diabetes.[22,23]

Hence, we can see that adipose tissue acts as much more than just a store for excess energy — it plays a major role in energy regulation and metabolism.

HYPOGONADISM AS AN ENDOCRINE DISEASE

Before we discuss obesity and its relationship with low testosterone, we will take a brief look at the physiology of normal gonadal function, and the pathophysiology of hypogonadism.

Testosterone is an essential anabolic steroid hormone that is secreted primarily by the testes, along with minor contribution from the adrenal glands.[24] Synthesis of this hormone is regulated through feedback control over the release of hypothalamic gonadotropin-releasing hormone (GnRH), which then stimulates the anterior pituitary gland to release gonadotropins, follicle-stimulating hormone, and luteinizing hormone, which in turn promote production and secretion of testosterone and help regulate spermatogenesis.[25] Testosterone, along with its 5-alpha reduction metabolite, dihydrotestosterone, exerts is effects via activation of the androgen receptor as well as via activation of the estrogen receptor by its aromatization metabolite, estradiol (E2). The majority of circulating testosterone is bound to proteins, mostly to sex hormone binding globulin (SHBG) and to a lesser extent serum albumin. Only a very small fraction of testosterone (about 1%–2%) is unbound, or "free," and thus biologically active and able to enter a cell and activate its receptor.[26] Upon binding to the androgen receptor, testosterone functions to regulate mitochondrial activity, increasing mitochondrial number, activating respiratory chain components, and increasing transcription of genes responsible for oxidative phosphorylation.[27]

Hypogonadism in men refers to a diminished functional activity of the testes that results in diminished testosterone production and secretion. Hypogonadism can be subdivided into primary and secondary hypogonadism, according to whether the defect is inherent within the testes or lies outside of the testes, respectively.[28] Primary hypogonadism is much less common, and is typically owing to hypofunction of the testes in the presence of normal function and anatomy of the hypothalamus and anterior pituitary. Causes of primary hypogonadism include injury, hemochromatosis, infections, and genetic disorders, such as Klinefelter syndrome. Secondary hypogonadism is much more common, and may be caused by a variety of different conditions, such as brain tumors, pituitary tumors, trauma, medication/drug toxicity, and other disease processes. For the past few decades, obesity has also become recognized an important cause of secondary hypogonadism.

INTERPLAY BETWEEN OBESITY AND LOW TESTOSTERONE

Among the numerous comorbidities associated with obesity, it has long been recognized that there is a strong association between obesity and low testosterone levels. In fact, reductions in testosterone levels correlate with the severity of obesity and men with a body mass index of greater than 35 to 40 kg/m^2 have more than a 50% reduction in total and free testosterone levels compared with lean men.[29] There are many different ways to look at the effects of androgens on adipose tissue and obesity, because the relationship is complicated and seems to be bidirectional.

Effects of Fat on Androgens

It is accepted that obesity-related decreases in total testosterone levels are primarily owing to reductions in SHBG, which are driven by obesity-associated hyperinsulinemia. Low SHBG has also been found to be a strong independent predictor of type 2 diabetes.[30] The degree of causality, however, is unclear. It has also become apparent as of late that there are a number of other factors involved in the interplay between obesity and hypogonadism, including the proinflammatory cytokines and hormones that are released by adipocytes.

We have alluded to some of the effects of adipose tissue (and hence, obesity) on testosterone. Specifically, higher levels of adiposity can lead to increased conversion of testosterone into estrogen, and deactivation of dihydrotestosterone, both of which may decrease circulating levels of androgens. This may then further lower the level of circulating testosterone, as the estrogens produced act as a negative feedback to the hypothalamic–pituitary axis, and suppress GnRH, thereby leading to lower luteinizing hormone levels and thus lower levels of testosterone released by the gonads. Additionally, as discussed, TNF-alpha and IL-6 have similar mechanisms of inhibiting GnRH secretion in the hypothalamus, and, thus, higher levels of adiposity will lead to lower testicular stimulation of testosterone release.[31]

Leptin also plays a role in the maintenance of circulating testosterone levels, likely through the interaction of intermediary proteins known as kiss-peptins and their effect on GnRH secretion. Because obese individuals often become insensitive to increased endogenous leptin production and develop a functional leptin resistance, the hypothalamus may lose this stimulation mechanism in this population. In fact, there is evidence that leptin therapy may restore gonadal function in morbidly obese individuals.[32]

We now understand that adipose tissue also produces enzymes that are involved in the metabolism of sex steroids. Although these proteins are produced primarily in the adrenal glands and gonads, adipose tissue contains enzymes that activate, inactivate, and convert steroid hormones as well.[33] The sheer mass of adipose tissue increases its relative contribution to steroid metabolism, and in premenopausal women, it can contribute up to 50% of their circulating estrogen, in the form of E2.

Obesity also can affect serum testosterone levels via its effect on SHBG. As discussed, the liver secretes SHBG into the blood where it binds testosterone with high affinity, regulating its bioavailability.[34] Changes in serum concentrations of SHBG thereby can alter the levels of free testosterone, effectively increasing or decreasing androgenic activity. Numerous factors have been implicated in both increasing or decreasing circulating SHBG levels, including obesity, as well as thyroid dysfunction, liver disease, and medications such as corticosteroids. Because of the direct effect of obesity on reducing circulating SHBG levels, it is important that the diagnosis of hypogonadism should depend on the measurement of free testosterone in this setting.[35]

Another important way in which obesity promotes hypogonadism is via its effect on sleep. Certainly obstructive sleep apnea, which is characterized by recurrent episodes of complete or partial obstruction of the upper airway during sleep, is an obvious and potentially dangerous effect of weight gain. The increase in both the prevalence and the severity of obesity has led to an increase in the prevalence of obstructive sleep apnea in recent years.[36,37] Obstructive sleep apnea, in turn is known to reduce circulating serum testosterone levels and, in fact, the degree is likely related to the severity of hypoxia during sleeping hours.[36] That said, that obesity is frequently associated with marked sleep disturbances, even when there is no evidence of obstructive sleep apnea.[38] In addition, the relationship between obesity and

sleep seems to be bidirectional; poor sleep has been implicated recently as a risk factor for the development of obesity and its complications. Although the exact mechanism is unclear, it seems to be mediated by alterations in concentrations of neuroendocrine modulators, including leptin and cortisol.[39]

Effects of Androgens on Fat

Studies have shown an inverse correlation between testosterone levels and the amount of visceral fat on an individual.[40] Patients with prostate cancer who are undergoing androgen deprivation therapy tend to show increased central obesity and higher percentages of body fat, as well as decreased amounts of lean muscle mass.[41] In turn, testosterone replacement has been shown to increase lean muscle mass.[42] In fact, decreasing lean muscle mass is a key feature of obesity, and in combination with the increase in fat mass, it can lead to increased mortality, especially in older men.[43] The effects of testosterone on increasing muscle mass are extremely well-documented.

The exact mechanism of testosterone's effect on adipose tissue is unclear, but there are a few proposed theories, such as by stimulating lipolysis, decreasing lipogenesis, and inhibiting lipid uptake. It has been speculated that this may occur through lipoprotein lipase, an enzyme that has been linked multiple times to obesity. Lipoprotein lipase increases the amount of fatty acids and fatty acid uptake, and has been shown to be inversely correlated with testosterone levels in sedentary obese men.[44] In addition to promoting obesity, testosterone deficiency may lead to dyslipidemia, with elevations of total cholesterol, low-density lipoprotein cholesterol, and triglycerides. However, this relationship is not entirely clear, and multiple studies seem to contradict one another, with some stating that testosterone deficiency is associated with higher low-density lipoprotein cholesterol and some finding no relationship at all.

With this observation, we can describe a vicious cycle. The metabolic syndrome suppresses testosterone biosynthesis, which in turn predisposes these men to the onset and development of metabolic syndrome (and obesity), thereby reinforcing the cycle.[45]

EFFECTS OF TREATMENT OF OBESITY ON TESTOSTERONE

Although there is an established correlative relationship between obesity and hypogonadism, it has recently also become evident that weight reduction can increase testosterone levels of obese men.[7] Furthermore, the degree of weight loss is proportional to the subsequent increase in testosterone. Researchers have proposed a number of mechanisms for this relationship.

As discussed, aromatase expressed by adipocytes is responsible for the conversion of testosterone to E2, thus lowering the circulating androgen concentration. It follows that a decrease in adipocyte mass, via a downregulation of aromatase activity, will thereby lead to an increase in the serum testosterone concentration. As well, the decrease in E2 in turn decreases negative feedback of E2 on the hypothalamus. GnRH and luteinizing hormone increase as a result, providing further support for testosterone synthesis in the gonad. This "virtuous" cycle of course can only occur in the patient with an intact hypothalamic–pituitary–gonadal axis.

A potential effect of weight loss on testosterone levels relates to the earlier summarized idea of adipose as an endocrine organ. This premise, referred to as the hypogonadal–obesity–adipokine hypothesis, suggests that a decrease in adipose mass will in turn reduce the inflammatory factors secreted by adipocytes, such as TNF-alpha and IL-6. This in turn reduces the inhibitory effect of these molecules on hypothalamic GnRH secretion, ultimately promoting an increase in the degree of testosterone production.[46]

Another proposed mechanism of improvement of testosterone levels after weight loss is via changes in SHBG. Even minor weight loss (<15% over 4.4 years) is associated with modest increases in total testosterone. Free testosterone levels, however, did not change in the same population, likely owing to the trend toward normalization of SHBG levels.[47] Again, it is important for this reason to stress measurement of both total and free testosterone levels as part of the evaluation of hypogonadism in the obese population.

Finally, as discussed, changes in sleep patterns can have dramatic effects on serum testosterone levels. Weight loss is known to reduce the risk of obstructive sleep apnea. In addition to this, major improvements in sleep quality, excessive daytime sleepiness, snoring, and nocturnal choking have all been observed after weight loss.[48] These improvements in sleep patterns after weight loss subsequently play a part in subsequent trends toward resolution of hypogonadism.

EFFECTS OF TREATMENT OF TESTOSTERONE ON OBESITY

Similar to the bidirectional relationship of obesity and hypogonadism, treating either of these conditions can subsequently help to treat the other. Just as weight loss helps to normalize testosterone levels and ameliorate the symptoms associated with hypogonadism, the normalizing of testosterone levels can help to promote weight loss. Significant improvement in body composition has been noted after testosterone therapy in multiple studies.[49]

Randomized controlled trials have shown beneficial effects of testosterone on body composition. In 1 study, a weekly administration of 100 mg IM of testosterone enanthate showed a significant increase in lean body mass and decline in serum cholesterol, and another study of 108 men over the age of 65 showed a net loss of 2.9 kg and increase in lean mass after testosterone treatment.[50,51] Additionally, testosterone administration to men with type 2 diabetes with testosterone deficiency led to a reduction of leptin, as well as a decrease in waist circumference and waist/hip ratio.[52] As with the effect of weight loss on testosterone levels, there are several theories regarding the relationship between testosterone therapy administration and the promotion of weight loss.

It has been proposed that the effect of testosterone on metabolic function may be related to its upregulation of multiple enzymes and transcription factors important to metabolic function, especially in mitochondria. The impairment of mitochondrial function in hypogonadism is believed to contribute to fatigue, insulin resistance, type 2 diabetes mellitus, cardiovascular disease, and the metabolic syndrome.[44] Testosterone may also have a positive effect on the lineage of mesenchymal pluripotent cells, shifting them from an adipogenic lineage to a myogenic lineage, thereby decreasing fat mass in favor of increased lean body mass.[53] Another, perhaps more simplistic albeit obvious way in which testosterone therapy leads to increased weight loss is via its positive effect on motivation and energy. Certainly, as demonstrated in other studies, this improvement of motivation can lead to an increased energy expenditure that may lead to sustained weight loss.[54]

SUMMARY

The relationship between obesity and hypogonadism is complicated. The relationship is bidirectional and there are numerous causative and correlative factors on both sides of the equation. Obesity is increasing in prevalence in epidemic proportions. Likewise, we are beginning to see the rapid increase in the incidence of male hypogonadism. It is only recently that we are learning the ways in which these 2 conditions exacerbate each other, and we are only beginning to understand how by treating one of these conditions, we can help to treat the other as well.

REFERENCES

1. Ogden C, Carroll M, Kit B. Prevalence of childhood and adult obesity in the United States, 2011-2012. JAMA 2014;311(8):806–14.
2. World Health Organization. Obesity and overweight. WHO fact sheet. Geneva (Switzerland): World Health Organization; 2015.
3. Jensen MD, Ryan DH, Apovian CM, et al. Guideline for the management of overweight and obesity for adults. J Am Coll Cardiol 2014;63:2985–3023.
4. Shrager B, Jibara GA, Tabrizian P, et al. Resection of nonalcoholic steatohepatitis-associated hepatocellular carcinoma: a Western experience. Int J Surg Oncol 2012;2012:915128.
5. Lamm S. Fighting fat. Ann Arbor (MI): Spry Publishing LLC; 2015.
6. Mulligan T, Frick MF, Zuraw QC, et al. Prevalence of hypogonadism in males aged at least 45 years: the HIM study. Int J Clin Pract 2006;60:762–9.
7. Corona G, Rastrelli G, Monami M, et al. Body weight loss reverts obesity–associated hypogonadotropic hypogonadism: a systematic review and meta-analysis. Eur J Endocrinol 2013;168:829–43.
8. Lunenfeld B, Mskhalaya G, Zitzmann M, et al. Recommendations on the diagnosis, treatment and monitoring of hypogonadism in men. Aging Male 2015;18(1):5–15.
9. Kapoor D, Malkin CJ, Channer KS, et al. Androgens, insulin resistance and vascular disease in men. Clin Endocrinol 2005;63:239–50.
10. Saad F, Haider A, Doros G, et al. Long-term treatment of hypogonadal men with testosterone produces substantial and sustained weight loss. Obesity (Silver Spring) 2013;21:1975–81.
11. Yassin A, Doros G. testosterone therapy in hypogonadal men results and sustained in a clinically meaningful weight loss. Clin Obes 2013;3: 73–83.
12. Kershaw EE, Flier JS. Adipose tissue as an endocrine organ. J Clin Endocrinol Metab 2004;89(6): 2548–56.
13. Fain JN, Madan AK, Hiler ML, et al. Comparison of the release of adipokines by adipose tissue, adipose tissue matrix, and adipocytes from visceral and subcutaneous abdominal adipose tissues of obese humans. Endocrinology 2004;145: 2273–82.
14. Zhang F, Basinski MB, Beals JM, et al. Crystal structure of the obese protein leptin-E100. Nature 1997; 387(6629):206–9.
15. Ramíreza S, Clareta Volume M. Hypothalamic ER stress: a bridge between leptin resistance and obesity. FEBS Lett 2015;589(14):1678–87.
16. Fernandez-Real JM, Ricart W. Insulin resistance and chronic cardiovascular inflammatory syndrome. Endocr Rev 2003;24:278–301.
17. López-Jaramillo P, Gómez-Arbeláez D, López-López J, et al. The role of leptin/adiponectin ratio in metabolic syndrome and diabetes. Horm Mol Biol Clin Investig 2014;18(1):37–45.
18. Friedman JM, Halaas JL. Leptin and the regulation of body weight in mammals. Nature 1998; 395:763–70.
19. Moreno-Eutimio MA, Acosta-Altamirano G. Immunometabolism of exercise and sedentary lifestyle. Cir Cir 2014;82(3):344–51.
20. Balsan GA, Vieira JL, Oliveira AM, et al. Relationship between adiponectin, obesity and insulin resistance. Rev Assoc Med Bras 2015;61(1):72–80.
21. ORourke RW, Metcalf MD, White AE, et al. Depot-specific differences in inflammatory mediators and a role for NK cells and IFN-gamma in inflammation in human adipose tissue. Int J Obes (Lond) 2009; 33(9):978–90.
22. Pischon T, Boeing H, Hoffmann K, et al. General and abdominal adiposity and risk of death in Europe. N Engl J Med 2008;359:2105–20.
23. Misra A, Garg A, Abate N, et al. Relationship of anterior and posterior subcutaneous abdominal fat to insulin sensitivity in nondiabetic men. Obes Res 1997; 5:93–9.
24. Mooradian AD, Morley JE, Korenman SG. Biological actions of androgens. Endocr Rev 1987;8(1):1–28.
25. Morales ABJ, Gooren LJ, Guay AT, et al. Endocrine aspects of mens sexual dysfunction. In: Lue TF, Basson R, Rosen R, et al, editors. Sexual medicine, sexual dysfunctions in men and women, 2nd international consultation on sexual dysfunctions. Paris (France): Paris Health Publications; 2004. p. 347–82.
26. Pinzone J. Principles and practice of endocrinology and metabolism. Philadelphia: Lippincott Williams & Wilkins; 2001. Available at: https://books.google.com/books?id=FVfzRvaucq8C&q=testosterone#v=snippet&q=hypogonadism&f=false. Accessed August 4, 2012.
27. Traish AM, Abdullah B, Yu G. Androgen deficiency and mitochondrial dysfunction: implications for fatigue, muscle dysfunction, insulin resistance, diabetes, and cardiovascular disease. Horm Mol Biol Clin Investig 2011;8:431–44.
28. Rivas A, Mulkey Z, Lado-Abeal J, et al. Diagnosing and managing low serum testosterone. Proc (Bayl Univ Med Cent) 2014;27(4):321–32.
29. Allan CA, McLachlan RI. Androgens and obesity. Curr Opin Endocrinol Diabetes Obes 2010;17:224–32.
30. Bhasin S, Cunningham GR, Hayes FJ, et al. Testosterone therapy in men with androgen deficiency syndromes: an Endocrine Society clinical practice guideline. J Clin Endocrinol Metab 2010;95(6): 2536–59.

31. Grossmann M, Gianatti EJ, Zajac JD. Testosterone and type 2 diabetes. Curr Opin Endocrinol Diabetes Obes 2010;17:247–56.

32. Licinio J, Caglayan S, Ozata M, et al. Phenotypic effects of leptin replacement on morbid obesity, diabetes mellitus, hypogonadism, and behavior in leptin-deficient adults. Proc Natl Acad Sci U S A 2004;101(13):4531–6.

33. Belanger C, Luu-The V, Dupont P, et al. Adipose tissue intracrinology: potential importance of local androgen/estrogen metabolism in the regulation of adiposity. Horm Metab Res 2002;34:737–45.

34. Hammond GL, Bocchinfuso WP. Sex hormone-binding globulin: gene organization and structure/function analyses. Horm Res 1996;45(3–5):197–201.

35. Simó R, Sáez-López C, Barbosa-Desongles A, et al. Novel insights in SHBG regulation and clinical implications. Trends Endocrinol Metab 2015; 26(7):376–83.

36. Lee W, Nagubadi S, Kryger MH, et al. Epidemiology of obstructive sleep apnea: a population-based perspective. Expert Rev Respir Med 2008;2:349–64.

37. Pelusi C, Pasquali R. Testosterone levels in obese male patients with obstructive sleep apnea syndrome: relation to oxygen desaturation, body weight, fat distribution and the metabolic parameters. J Endocrinol Invest 2003;26(6):493–8.

38. Resta O, Foschino-Barbaro MP, Legari G, et al. Sleep-related breathing disorders, loud snoring and excessive daytime sleepiness in obese subjects. Int J Obes Relat Metab Disord 2001;25(5): 669–75.

39. Beccutia G, Pannaina S. Sleep and obesity. Curr Opin Clin Nutr Metab Care 2011;14(4):402–12.

40. Tsai EC, Boko EJ, Leonetti DL, et al. Low serum testosterone level as a predictor of increased visceral fat in Japanese-American men. Int J Obes Relat Metab Disord 2000;24:485–91.

41. Mauras N, Hayes V, Welch S, et al. Testosterone deficiency in young men: marked alterations in whole body protein kinetics, strength, and adiposity. J Clin Endocrinol Metab 1998;83:1886–92.

42. Hoyes CM, Yee BJ, Philllips CL, et al. Body compositional and cardiometabolic effects of testosterone therapy in obese men with severe obstructive sleep apnoea: a randomized placebo-controlled trial. Eur J Endocrinol 2012;167:531–41.

43. Lee CG, Boyko EJ, Nelson CM, et al. Mortality risk in older men associated with changes in weight, lean mass, and fat mass. J Am Geriatr Soc 2011;59: 233–40.

44. Ramirez ME, McMurry MP, Wiebje GA, et al. Evidence for sex steroid inhibition of lipoprotein lipase in men: comparison of abdominal and femoral adipose tissue. Metabolism 1997;46:179–85.

45. Stellato RK, Feldman HA, Hamdy O, et al. Testosterone, sex hormone-binding globulin, and the development of type 2 diabetes in middle-aged men: prospective results from the Massachusetts male aging study. Diabetes Care 2000;23(4):490–4.

46. Jones TH. Testosterone association with erectile dysfunction, diabetes, and the metabolic syndrome. Eur Urol 2007;6:847–57.

47. Ng Tang Fui M, Dupuis P, Grossmann M. Lowered testosterone in male obesity: mechanisms, morbidity and management. Asian J Androl 2014; 16(2):223–31.

48. Dixon J, Schachter L, O'Brien P. Sleep disturbance and obesity: changes following surgically induced weight loss. Arch Intern Med 2001;161:102–6.

49. Saad F, Aversa A, Isidori AM, et al. Testosterone as potential effective therapy in treatment of obesity in men with testosterone deficiency: a review. Curr Diabetes Rev 2012;8:131–43.

50. Mårin P, Holmäng S, Gustafsson C, et al. Androgen treatment of abdominally obese men. Obes Res 1993;1(4):245–51.

51. Snyder PJ, Peachey H, Hannoush P, et al. Effect of testosterone treatment on body composition and muscle strength in men over 65 years of age. J Clin Endocrinol Metab 1999;84(8):2647–53.

52. Kapoor D, Clarke S, Stanworth R, et al. The effect of testosterone replacement therapy on adipocytokines and C-reactive protein in hypogonadal men with type 2 diabetes. Eur J Endocrinol 2007;156(5): 595–602.

53. Singh R, Artaza JN, Taylor WE, et al. Androgens stimulate myogenic differentiation and inhibit adipogenesis in C3H 10T1/2 pluripotent cells through an androgen receptor-mediated pathway. Endocrinology 2003;144:5081–8.

54. Sattler F, Bhasin S, He J, et al. Testosterone threshold levels and lean tissue mass targets needed to enhance skeletal muscle strength and function: the HORMA trial. J Gerontol A Biol Sci Med Sci 2011;66:122–9.

Management of Hypogonadism in Cardiovascular Patients

What Are the Implications of Testosterone Therapy on Cardiovascular Morbidity?

Monique S. Tanna, MD[a], Arthur Schwartzbard, MD[b],
Jeffery S. Berger, MD[b], James Underberg, MD[b],
Eugenia Gianos, MD[b], Howard S. Weintraub, MD[b,*]

KEYWORDS

- Testosterone • Androgens • Cardiovascular risk • Mortality • Hypogonadism
- Androgen deficiency

KEY POINTS

- Testosterone replacement therapy should only be prescribed to men with both clinical symptoms of androgen deficiency and unequivocally low testosterone levels.
- Despite a relatively constant prevalence of male hypogonadism, there has been a striking increase in testosterone prescription without adequate diagnosis or monitoring.
- Recent studies have raised concern regarding a potential increase in cardiovascular events with testosterone therapy; however, these are mostly retrospective analyses with considerable limitations.
- As with most hormonal therapies, it is likely that both low and high levels cause adverse outcomes, making it critical to monitor on-treatment testosterone levels.
- Testosterone therapy can be safely considered in men with cardiovascular disease and appropriately diagnosed symptomatic hypogonadism after a thorough discussion of potential risks and with guideline-recommended safety monitoring.

INTRODUCTION

Testosterone replacement therapy is recommended for the treatment of men with established clinical androgen deficiency. Also known as male hypogonadism, the diagnosis of clinical androgen deficiency requires both clinical signs and symptoms of androgen deficiency as well as unequivocally low morning testosterone levels.[1] Despite a relatively constant prevalence of hypogonadism, there has been a dramatic increase in testosterone prescription in both the United States and the United Kingdom in recent years suggesting inappropriate therapy. In the United States, testosterone prescription among men 40 years of age and older has increased more than 3-fold from 0.81% in 2001 to 2.91% in 2011.[2] Most of these men did not have an apparent indication for therapy, and more than 25% did not have testosterone levels measured in the prior 12 months.[2] General awareness of testosterone deficiency has also increased as evidenced by a 137% increase in

a Division of Cardiology, New York University School of Medicine, 462 First Avenue, NBV 17 South, New York, NY 10016, USA; b Division of Cardiology, New York University School of Medicine, New York, NY, USA
* Corresponding author. 530 First Avenue, Suite 4F, New York, NY 10016.
E-mail address: howard.weintraub@nyumc.org

Urol Clin N Am 43 (2016) 247–260
http://dx.doi.org/10.1016/j.ucl.2016.01.011
0094-0143/16/$ – see front matter © 2016 Elsevier Inc. All rights reserved.

Clinical case

A 53-year-old man with a history of tobacco use, obesity, hyperlipidemia, glucose intolerance, and obstructive sleep apnea (OSA) was diagnosed with hypogonadism. He was started on intramuscular testosterone injections, and his total testosterone level increased to 1130 ng/dL with an improvement in symptoms. He underwent screening coronary calcium score assessment, which was found to be elevated with a score of 655, most of which localized to the right coronary artery. The patient was only able to tolerate a maximum of 10 mg of rosuvastatin daily because of myalgias. The following year, he developed severe chest discomfort while exercising and sustained an inferior wall myocardial infarction. He underwent percutaneous coronary intervention with stent placement to the right coronary artery. Testosterone supplementation was discontinued at that time. His current morning testosterone level is 249 ng/dL, and he reports symptoms of fatigue and decreased libido.

1. Should this patient's supplemental testosterone have been discontinued earlier in light of his elevated calcium score and significant cardiovascular risk factors?
2. What are the risks, benefits, and contraindications of testosterone supplementation and how should patients be monitored?
3. Does testosterone therapy increase the risk of cardiovascular morbidity and mortality?
4. Can this patient be safely restarted on testosterone therapy?

the number of men requesting serum testosterone evaluation,[3] likely due to increased marketing of testosterone therapy for *low T syndrome* targeting elderly men with sexual dysfunction and fatigue.

Concurrently, the role of testosterone therapy in cardiovascular morbidity and mortality has become the topic of vigorous debate. Recently published retrospective analyses have raised concern regarding the potential adverse cardiovascular effects of testosterone therapy, challenging the longstanding premise that treatment of hypogonadism with testosterone therapy not only mitigates the symptoms of hypogonadism but also its associated increase in mortality. In this review, the authors discuss the findings and validity of these recent studies as well as their implications on the treatment of hypogonadism in cardiovascular patients.

NATURAL HISTORY OF TESTOSTERONE LEVELS

Male hypogonadism affects a large number of middle-aged and older men and not only impairs quality of life but also overall morbidity and mortality. The Massachusetts Male Aging Study estimated the prevalence of clinical androgen deficiency to be 12.3% (2.4 million individuals) among men aged 40 to 69 years in the United States with an annual incidence of 481,000 new cases per year.[4] Studies have shown an average age-related decline in testosterone levels of 1% to 2% per year,[1] resulting in an increasing prevalence of testosterone deficiency with age, estimated at 20% in men older than 60 years, 30% in men older than 70 years, and 50% in men older than 80 years.[5]

This decline is thought to be due to defects in both testicular and hypothalamic-pituitary function. Additionally, levels of sex hormone–binding globulin (SHBG) increase with age, resulting in a greater percentage of bound testosterone and thereby less bioavailable testosterone.[5–7] Bioavailable testosterone consists of serum-free testosterone (1%–2% of total testosterone) and albumin-bound testosterone, which readily dissociates in tissue transit (approximately 40% of total testosterone).[8] The remaining 50% to 60% is strongly bound to SHBG and not bioavailable.

CLINICAL DIAGNOSIS AND MANAGEMENT OF HYPOGONADISM

Not all men with low testosterone levels have clinical androgen deficiency or hypogonadism, however; this clinical diagnosis must be made in accordance with the Endocrine Society's practice guideline.[1] The diagnosis of clinical androgen deficiency requires both clinical signs and symptoms of testosterone deficiency as well as an unequivocally low testosterone level based on the reference range for the specific assay used and established in each laboratory (usually 280–300 ng/dL).[1] In older men aged 65 to 80 years, some experts recommend the same cutoff of 300 ng/dL, whereas others recommend a more stringent cutoff of 200 ng/dL based on the lack of benefit of testosterone replacement therapy seen in older men with pretreatment testosterone values of 300 ng/dL.[1] Furthermore, because testosterone peaks in the morning because of circadian variation, testosterone levels must be measured in the morning. They should also be collected in the absence of subacute or acute illness and be confirmed by at least one repeat measurement. Free or bioavailable testosterone levels should only be used when total testosterone is near the lower limit of normal and alteration in SHBG is suspected, such as in patients with obesity, diabetes mellitus, liver disease, thyroid disease, nephrotic syndrome, advanced age, and chronic illness.

Before initiation of testosterone replacement therapy, patients should be evaluated for causes of secondary hypogonadism based on clinical suspicion, including hyperprolactinemia, genetic disorders, hemochromatosis, and pituitary neoplasm among others.

Men with appropriately diagnosed clinical androgen deficiency should be treated with testosterone replacement therapy. There are various formulations and routes of administration available, with the topical gel formulation having had the greatest incline in use making it the most commonly prescribed formulation in current practice and representing 65% of testosterone prescriptions.[2,3,9]

Patients being treated with testosterone replacement therapy must be appropriately monitored with on-treatment hematocrit as well as testosterone levels, which should be in the midnormal range at 3 to 6 months and in older men in the lower part of the normal range of young men (400–500 ng/dL).[1] Further detail on indications, contraindications, and administration of testosterone replacement therapy can be found elsewhere in this issue (See Burschtin O: Testosterone deficiency and sleep apnea, in this issue; Gannon JR, Walsh TJ: Testosterone and sexual function, in this issue).

WHAT ARE THE CLINICAL MANIFESTATIONS OF TESTOSTERONE DEFICIENCY?
Adverse Symptoms and Physiologic Consequences

Several cross-sectional and longitudinal studies have demonstrated the sexual, psychological, and physical consequences of untreated testosterone deficiency. Low testosterone levels are associated with reduced sexual interest, sexual activity, and libido[10–13]; loss of bone mineral density and increased fracture risk[12,14–16]; decreased muscle mass and strength[15]; increased fat mass[15]; fatigue and depressed mood[13,17,18]; and a decline in cognitive function.[19]

Increase in Metabolic Syndrome and Other Cardiovascular Risk Factors

Low testosterone levels are also associated with increased risk of the individual components of the metabolic syndrome, including insulin resistance and subsequent type II diabetes mellitus,[20–24] central adiposity,[25,26] increased triglycerides, total cholesterol and low-density lipoprotein levels,[27,28] and decreased high-density lipoprotein levels.[29,30] Furthermore, several cross-sectional and longitudinal studies have shown that testosterone deficiency is associated with an increased risk of the metabolic syndrome.[21,25] The Massachusetts Male Aging Study prospectively followed 950 men aged 40 to 70 years for 15 years and found a 2- to 4-fold increase in the risk of metabolic syndrome in men with a body mass index less than 25 who were in the lowest quartile of total testosterone ($\leq$415 ng/dL) compared with those in the highest quartile (>628 ng/dL).[31] Testosterone deficiency has also been shown to be associated with several cardiovascular risk factors, including increased carotid intimal media thickness,[32–34] peripheral arterial disease,[35] and elevated high-sensitivity C-reactive protein.[36]

Increased All-Cause and Cardiovascular Mortality

Testosterone deficiency is associated with an increase in both all-cause mortality and cardiovascular mortality. A large prospective cohort study of 3014 Swedish men aged 69 to 80 years followed for 4.5 years found that men in the lowest quartile of total testosterone ($\leq$97 ng/dL) had an increased mortality (hazard ratio [HR] 1.65) compared with those in the other 3 quartiles.[37] Another prospective cohort study of 794 men aged 50 to 91 years (mean age 71 years) followed for 11.8 years also showed not only increased mortality (HR 1.40) but also an increased risk of both cardiovascular (HR 1.38) and respiratory disease (HR 2.29) among men with the lowest quartile of total testosterone (<241 ng/dL).[38] A prospective population-based study of almost 2000 men aged 20 to 79 years in Pomerania also found an association between low testosterone levels (<250 ng/dL) and both all-cause mortality (HR 2.32) and cardiovascular mortality (HR 2.56).[39] Several subsequent studies and meta-analyses have similarly shown an association between testosterone deficiency and both all-cause mortality[40,41] and cardiovascular mortality,[41–45] including in a subpopulation of men with known coronary disease.[46]

Although some prospective trials of younger men (mean age early 50s) failed to show an association between testosterone deficiency and mortality, they instead showed an increased risk of ischemic heart disease.[47,48] Other meta-analyses have shown only an increase in cardiovascular risk in elderly men with low testosterone levels,[49] postulating that testosterone deficiency may simply be a marker of poor underlying health status.[45,49] Although the evidence is conflicting, several studies have found increased cardiovascular morbidity and mortality in men being treated for prostate cancer with androgen deprivation therapy (ADT). Although it is unknown whether this increased risk is limited to those with preexisting coronary artery disease,[50,51] there are substantial data demonstrating the adverse effects of ADT on traditional cardiovascular risk factors, such as serum lipoproteins, insulin sensitivity, and obesity.[51]

EFFECTS OF TESTOSTERONE REPLACEMENT THERAPY: PROSPECTIVE DATA
Improvement in Symptoms and Components of the Metabolic Syndrome

Several studies have shown that testosterone replacement therapy in men with clinical androgen deficiency improves sexual function and libido, increases lean body mass and physical function, increases bone mineral density, decreases depression scores, and improves mood and quality of life.[52–63] Although mostly small studies, several randomized controlled trials of testosterone therapy in men with testosterone deficiency and type II diabetes mellitus or metabolic syndrome have shown improvement in various components of the metabolic syndrome, including atherogenic dyslipidemia, insulin resistance, glycemic control, and inflammatory markers, including c-reactive protein levels.[64–67] A meta-analysis of 20 cross-sectional, longitudinal, and randomized studies further showed that testosterone replacement therapy is associated with both improved metabolic control and central obesity.[68] Whether the improvement in metabolic syndrome and its individual components is a direct effect of testosterone therapy or the result of the concurrent reduction in abdominal obesity seen in many of these studies is unknown.

Improvement in Cardiac Functional Capacity

Randomized controlled trials of testosterone therapy have shown improvement in functional capacity in both men with coronary disease as well as those with chronic heart failure. A double-blind, randomized, placebo-controlled study of 46 men with stable angina treated with low-dose transdermal testosterone versus placebo showed a delay in time to 1-mm ST-segment depression on treadmill exercise testing in the testosterone arm consistent with reduced exercise-induced myocardial ischemia.[69] Those with lower baseline testosterone levels had a greater magnitude of

this response. In those receiving testosterone therapy, testosterone levels increased from 390 ng/dL at baseline to 644 ng/dL at 6 weeks and 535 ng/dL at 14 weeks. Another randomized placebo-controlled study showed similar improvement in myocardial ischemia with testosterone replacement therapy and a sustained effect at 12 months.[70]

Similarly, randomized placebo-controlled trials of testosterone therapy in men with heart failure have demonstrated that low testosterone levels correlate with reduced functional capacity as assessed by both the incremental shuttle walk test (ISWT) and peak oxygen consumption (Vo_2).[71,72] Although guideline recommendations advise against treating men with uncontrolled or poorly controlled heart failure with testosterone therapy, these randomized controlled trials were conducted in men with stable heart failure and a moderately reduced ejection fraction and showed that testosterone therapy improves objective functional capacity based on the ISWT and peak Vo_2 as well as symptomatic functional class without an increase in cardiovascular events, hospital admissions, or mortality.[71,72]

Progression of Atherosclerotic Risk Factors

A recent randomized placebo-controlled trial of 308 men aged 60 years or older (mean age 67.6 years) with low to low-normal testosterone levels showed no change in the surrogate end points of carotid artery intima-media thickness and coronary artery calcium with the use of testosterone gel versus placebo gel over 3 years.[73] Furthermore, there was no difference in secondary outcomes of sexual function or health-related quality of life. Of note, the mean baseline total testosterone level was 307 ng/dL in both groups, and approximately a third of patients had testosterone levels between 300 and 400 ng/dL. Interestingly, the lower limit of normal reference range for the specific assay used to measure testosterone in this study is 250 ng/dL in men aged 18 to 69 years, which is lower than the 300 to 320 ng/dL cutoff used in most assays.[74] Furthermore, in men aged 70 to 89 years, the lower limit of normal for this assay is 90 ng/dL. This finding suggests that at least a third, if not more, of enrolled patients did not have clinical hypogonadism as defined by the Endocrine Society's guidelines summarized earlier. The average testosterone level at which symptoms of androgen deficiency occur in most studies corresponds to the lower limit of normal range for young men, which is approximately 300 ng/dL.[1] However, normal ranges vary depending on the assay and laboratory; clinicians are advised to use the lower limit of normal that has been established in their laboratory.[1]

Indeed, the authors agree that some men in the trial had low-normal testosterone levels and that participants were not selected based on a diagnosis of hypogonadism or clinical symptoms of hypogonadism as is often the case in current clinical practice. This trial failed to show not only a reduction in atherosclerotic risk factors with testosterone therapy but also failed to show an improvement in sexual function or quality of life, contrary to most studies of testosterone replacement. This failure is likely explained by the fact that many participants did not have clinical androgen deficiency as defined by the Endocrine Society's guideline and further supports the recommendation that testosterone therapy should only be administered to those men with appropriately diagnosed hypogonadism.

Signal Toward Increased Cardiovascular Events

Several recent studies suggesting that testosterone replacement therapy may be associated with an increase in cardiovascular events prompted the Endocrine Society to issue a statement regarding this potential risk and reinforcing that testosterone prescription should only be administered to men with appropriately diagnosed clinical androgen deficiency and with adequate safety monitoring.[75]

The Testosterone in Older Men with Mobility Limitations (TOM) trial was a prospective, randomized placebo-controlled study to determine the effects of testosterone gel versus placebo gel on lower extremity strength and physical function in 209 men older than 65 years (mean age 74 years) with low total testosterone (100–350 ng/dL) or free testosterone (<50 pg/mL) levels and limitations in mobility.[76] A higher incidence of cardiovascular signs or symptoms that were not prespecified was observed in the testosterone group, leading to early termination of the trial. It is important to consider several factors when interpreting this study. First, the cardiovascular events found in this study were not predefined and included a wide variety of signs and symptoms, including some of unclear clinical significance, such as self-reported tachycardia with fatigue, peripheral edema, left ventricular strain pattern during exercise testing, and ectopy noted on electrocardiogram. Additionally, the study was not designed to evaluate cardiovascular outcomes but rather the effects of testosterone on muscle function. Furthermore, both the small number of total

adverse events and early termination of the trial may have led to an overestimation of treatment differences.

Along with the methodological issues in interpreting these results, there were also multiple confounders that could have played a role in the study results. The testosterone gel dose used in this study was a higher off-label dosage of 100 mg per day, whereas the recommended initial dosage is 50 mg daily. Testosterone levels increased from 243 ng/dL to 574 ±403 ng/dL in the testosterone group, with some subjects achieving testosterone levels well more than the recommended midnormal range. Indeed, there was an increased risk of cardiovascular events in men in the highest quartile of on-treatment testosterone level (512–1957 ng/dL) compared with all other subjects (HR 2.4, $P = .05$), which may partly be explained by supratherapeutic testosterone levels in these patients. Additionally, the study population was a higher risk older population with a high prevalence of hypertension, hyperlipidemia, diabetes, and obesity at baseline; there was a higher prevalence of patients on antihypertensive and statin therapy in the testosterone arm. Within the testosterone arm, those who experienced cardiovascular events had lower testosterone levels at baseline, suggesting a greater underlying disease burden.[77]

An increased risk of cardiovascular events was also seen in a meta-analysis of 27 small, randomized placebo-controlled trials consisting of 2994 older men treated with at least 12 weeks of testosterone therapy (odds ratio [OR] 1.54, 95% confidence interval [CI] 1.09–2.18).[78] Interestingly, this effect varied with the source of funding but not with baseline testosterone levels. The risk of cardiovascular events was lower in the 13 pharmaceutical industry funded trials compared with those that were not industry sponsored (OR 0.89 vs 2.06). Industry-funded trials had younger subjects and used different definitions of cardiovascular events as well as different reporting of adverse effects, which may have contributed to this observed difference.

Studies Showing No Effect on Cardiovascular Events

Several randomized trials and meta-analyses have shown that testosterone replacement therapy is not associated with an increase in cardiovascular events, although most are small heterogeneous studies of variable duration.[62,79–82] A recently published and now the largest meta-analysis of 75 placebo-controlled randomized trials of testosterone therapy including 3016 testosterone-treated patients and 2448 placebo-treated found no association between testosterone therapy and cardiovascular risk and additionally showed a reduction in body fat and increase in lean muscle mass with testosterone replacement therapy.[83]

Reduction in Mortality

A longitudinal cohort study by Muraleedharan and colleagues[84] prospectively followed 581 men with type 2 diabetes for a mean of 41.6 months and found that the 238 men with low total testosterone levels (≤300 ng/dL) had increased mortality rates (17.2% vs 9.0%, HR 2.02, 95% CI 1.2–3.4) compared with the 343 who did not. Those who were treated with testosterone replacement were appropriately diagnosed with clinical androgen deficiency and achieved guideline-recommended on-treatment testosterone levels (mean peak on-treatment level 657 ng/dL). Of the 238 men with low total testosterone levels, the 64 who were treated had reduced mortality (8.4% vs 19.2%, adjusted HR 2.3, 95% CI 1.3–3.9), suggesting that testosterone replacement therapy in these men improves survival. Although this was not a randomized trial, the major strength of this study is that all patients were appropriately diagnosed, treated, and monitored per guideline recommendations.

EFFECTS OF TESTOSTERONE REPLACEMENT THERAPY: RETROSPECTIVE DATA
Potential Increase in Cardiovascular Events and Mortality

There have been a few recent retrospective studies suggesting increased cardiovascular events and mortality with testosterone therapy. A retrospective cohort study of 8709 men who had undergone prior coronary angiography in the Veterans Affairs system and also had low testosterone levels (<300 ng/dL) found that the 1223 men who were prescribed testosterone therapy had increased risk of the composite end point of all-cause mortality, myocardial infarction, and ischemic stroke compared with the 7486 who were not (25.7% vs 19.9%, HR 1.29, 95% CI 1.04–1.58), and this was irrespective of the presence of prior coronary artery disease or revascularization.[85] Although compelling, further inspection reveals that this trial has several limitations, resulting in significant controversy.[86–90] There is an inherent selection bias in this study given that only 1223 men were prescribed testosterone therapy, despite the fact that all of the men in this cohort had low testosterone levels. The inclusion criteria of this study did not require a clinical diagnosis of hypogonadism; it is possible

that more men in the treated group had clinical androgen deficiency, which in itself is associated with higher mortality. Baseline testosterone levels were also lower in the treated group (175.5 vs 206.5 ng/dL), suggesting a greater severity of androgen deficiency and underlying disease burden.

Furthermore, there is no evidence that testosterone was prescribed or monitored as per the guidelines as only 60% of the treated group had repeat testosterone measurements; it is possible that treated patients may have been undertreated or overtreated, both of which can be potentially harmful. Among those patients who did have a repeat measurement, the level was 332.2 ng/dL, which is lower than the recommended goal in the midnormal range, suggesting undertreatment. It is possible that the increased mortality seen in treated patients may reflect inadequate treatment in patients with more severe hypogonadism. Additionally, although the investigators reported a long-term duration of therapy, 18% of subjects had filled only one prescription.

A subsequent cohort study reported increased risk of nonfatal myocardial infarction (relative risk [RR] 1.36) among 55,593 individuals in a large health care database derived from insurance company records in the first 90 days after filling their first prescription of testosterone compared with the prior 1 year.[91] This association was observed in men aged 65 years and older (RR 2.19) and in younger men with preexisting heart disease (RR 2.90). Again, there were no data on follow-up testosterone levels or adequacy of treatment. Given that testosterone deficiency itself is associated with increased cardiovascular mortality, the observed increase in nonfatal myocardial infarction could be due to the underlying androgen deficiency rather than testosterone therapy.

Most recently, a retrospective cohort study comparing the cardiovascular safety of testosterone injections, patches, and gels in the United States and the United Kingdom using insurance claims data in men aged 18 years or older showed that testosterone injection users had a higher rate of cardiovascular events (myocardial infarction, unstable angina, and stroke; HR 1.26, 95% CI 1.18–1.35), hospitalization (HR 1.16, 95% CI 1.13–1.19) and death (HR 1.34, 95% CI 1.15–1.56) when compared with men using testosterone gel.[92] There was no difference in outcomes between men using testosterone gels and patches. The study did not include a comparator group of untreated men. It can be postulated that given the nonphysiologic peaks and troughs of testosterone injection, this formulation may lead to inappropriately high testosterone levels, which can potentially be harmful. However, as in other retrospective analyses, this study also did not assess the validity of testosterone prescription or whether these patients were diagnosed with clinical androgen deficiency. It also lacked data on testosterone levels both at initiation of therapy and during treatment. Furthermore, it is possible that those men prescribed testosterone injection were at a higher baseline cardiovascular risk than those prescribed testosterone gel as evidenced by the fact that the most Medicare patients, who were significantly older, were injection users, whereas most commercially insured US patients were gel users. Given these limitations, it is difficult to draw a conclusion on whether testosterone injections are truly associated with adverse events; further study is needed to evaluate this potential association.

Reduction in Mortality

A retrospective analysis of 1031 men (average age 62 years) with testosterone levels of 250 ng/dL or less from 7 Veterans Affairs medical centers found that the 398 men who were treated with testosterone replacement therapy had lower mortality than those who were untreated (10.3% vs 20.7%, adjusted HR 0.61, 95% CI 0.42–0.88).[93] This study also evaluated the duration of treatment rather than initial prescription only, which has been a limitation of some studies. In a secondary analysis whereby men who stopped treatment were censored at 90 days after their last treatment date also found that testosterone therapy was associated with a decrease in mortality. Furthermore, a correlation was seen between higher mortality and both lower baseline testosterone levels as well as a shorter duration of testosterone treatment, supporting that testosterone deficiency is associated with increased mortality and that testosterone replacement therapy in these patients is associated with improved survival.

Another limitation of recent studies suggesting an increase in cardiovascular events with testosterone therapy is the lack of on-treatment monitoring of testosterone levels to ensure adequate treatment and avoid supraphysiologic testosterone levels. To address this concern, Sharma and colleagues[94] performed a retrospective analysis of 83,010 men in the Veterans Affairs system (median age 66 years) with low testosterone levels and analyzed outcomes based on whether subjects received testosterone replacement prescriptions as well as whether follow-up testosterone levels were in the normal range. The 43,931 men who were treated with any form of testosterone replacement therapy and achieved normal follow-up testosterone levels (mean follow-up 6.2 years) were compared with the 13,378 untreated men (mean follow-up 4.7 years) and were found to have significantly lower rates of all-cause mortality (HR 0.44, 95% CI 0.42–0.46), myocardial infarction (HR 0.76, 95% CI 0.63–0.93) and stroke (HR 0.64, 95% CI, 0.43–0.96). When this group of 43,391 men was compared with the 25,701 men receiving testosterone therapy without achieving normal follow-up testosterone levels (mean follow-up 4.6 years), they again showed significantly lower rates of all-cause mortality, myocardial infarction, and stroke. Compared with untreated men, the group of men who were treated but did not achieve normalization of follow-up testosterone levels showed decreased all-cause mortality (HR 0.84, 95% CI 0.80–0.89) but no difference in rates of myocardial infarction or stroke.

This study includes the largest cohort of patients with hypogonadism and demonstrates the critical role of follow-up testosterone levels on determining the benefits and adverse effects of testosterone therapy. The investigators showed that patients treated with testosterone therapy who achieve normalized testosterone levels indeed have lower rates of mortality as well as myocardial infarction. This study is one of the few studies to analyze outcomes with testosterone replacement therapy based on adequate treatment rather than treatment alone without data on follow-up testosterone levels, which has been a major limitation of previous studies. However, this study does have its own limitations, namely, the likelihood of unmeasured confounders among the 3 groups. Because of the nature of this retrospective analysis, there is no information on why some patients were treated with testosterone replacement, whereas others were not and, among those who were treated, why some did not achieve normalization of levels. Although it is reasonable to label this group as inadequately treated, it can be postulated that the differences observed in this group may be due to differences in baseline characteristics. For example, this group may have been sicker with lower testosterone levels at baseline and more severe hypogonadism; they may have been less motivated and/or noncompliant with testosterone therapy; or they may have received less medical follow-up, all of which can contribute to poorer outcomes. Similarly, it is also unknown why the untreated group was not treated with testosterone therapy and again may have had unmeasured differences in baseline characteristics, such as more severe hypogonadism, greater number of comorbidities precluding treatment with testosterone therapy, and so on, which may have contributed to the reported outcomes. Although the investigators used propensity score-weighted Cox proportional hazard models, the 3 groups were significantly different at baseline and the presence of unmeasured confounders is likely.

WHAT ROLE DOES TESTOSTERONE PLAY IN CARDIOVASCULAR DISEASE AND ITS RISK FACTORS AND WHAT ARE THE POTENTIAL MECHANISMS?

There are various mechanisms by which testosterone may play a role in cardiovascular disease and its risk factors. As discussed earlier, observational studies have shown worsening of the metabolic syndrome and its risk factors in testosterone deficiency and an improvement in these with testosterone supplementation. The beneficial effects of testosterone therapy on cardiovascular mortality and outcomes seen in some studies may be explained by a potential improvement in cardiovascular risk factors; however, this has not been studied and requires further elucidation.

The prospective randomized TOM trial used an off-label higher dose of testosterone replacement therapy, achieving testosterone levels well more than the recommended midnormal range; men in the highest quartile of testosterone levels (512–1957 ng/dL) had a greater increase in cardiovascular events.[76] Similarly, the retrospective analyses discussed earlier that showed an increase in cardiovascular events with testosterone therapy did not assess on-treatment testosterone levels. Given the likelihood of inappropriate therapy in current practice as evidenced by increased marketing for *low T syndrome* and an increase in testosterone therapy without appropriate diagnosis or follow-up, it can be postulated that many of these adverse effects may in fact be the result of inappropriate therapy or inadequate monitoring, both of which may result in inappropriately high testosterone levels. As with any hormone, it is likely that both low and high levels can have adverse consequences.

There are several mechanisms by which supranormal testosterone levels may be harmful. A small fraction (5%–10%) of testosterone is metabolized to dihydrotestosterone, which increases expression of vascular cell adhesion molecule-1 and promotes monocyte adhesion to the vascular endothelium in a dose-dependent manner, resulting in progression of atherosclerosis.[95,96] Dihydrotestosterone has been shown to be associated with incident cardiovascular disease and all-cause mortality with increased risk at both low and high levels in a longitudinal study of elderly men without baseline cardiovascular disease.[97] Furthermore, intramuscular testosterone injections lead to increased platelet thromboxane A2 receptor density stimulating platelet aggregation, with return to baseline after cessation of therapy.[98] Platelet aggregation plays a key role in thrombus formation and can increase the risk of acute plaque rupture.

Inadequate safety monitoring of hemoglobin and hematocrit levels as required by guidelines can also lead to adverse outcomes given that exogenous testosterone increases these levels[58,76,80–82] and is the most frequent adverse effect of testosterone therapy. We know from studies of patients with polycythemia vera that those who have more intensive hematocrit lowering have lower cardiovascular risk, suggesting that polycythemia itself is a risk factor for cardiovascular events.[99] Testosterone therapy can also worsen sleep-disordered breathing in men with severe OSA[100] and is, therefore, contraindicated in untreated patients.[1] OSA is a known risk factor for atherosclerosis and can contribute to the increase in cardiovascular events if men are not being appropriately screened before the initiation of testosterone therapy.

Additionally, testosterone is converted to estradiol via aromatase; there is a dose-dependent increase in estradiol levels with testosterone therapy.[101,102] Elevated estradiol levels are associated with coronary thrombosis,[103] peripheral arterial disease,[35] and stroke[104] and may be a mediator of adverse cardiovascular events. Although not statistically significant, men who experienced cardiovascular events in the TOM trial had estradiol levels that were twice as high as those who did not.[77] Estrogen administration in men has also been shown to increase the risk of thromboembolism and nonfatal myocardial infarction.[105]

Furthermore, many men are being inappropriately treated with testosterone without an adequate diagnosis and for inappropriate indications, such as erectile dysfunction. Men with erectile dysfunction share many risk factors with those who have cardiovascular disease, and studies suggest that erectile dysfunction is an independent risk marker for cardiovascular disease.[106,107] Erectile dysfunction in elderly men does not necessarily have a hormonal cause, and self-selection of these patients for testosterone therapy leads to selection bias and confounders that may explain the observed increase in cardiovascular events seen in this group.

Finally, there is an inherent limitation of retrospective studies given the necessary difference in baseline characteristics of men who are treated with testosterone replacement therapy versus those who are not resulting in an unavoidable selection bias. Even with sophisticated statistical analyses, the presence of unmeasured confounders is likely. It is possible that those who are treated are more likely to have clinical androgen deficiency with its associated symptoms and increased mortality, whereas those who are not treated may have low testosterone levels that are clinically insignificant.

WHAT ARE OTHER THERAPEUTIC OPTIONS FOR CLINICAL ANDROGEN DEFICIENCY?

Given that aromatase converts testosterone to estradiol, excess aromatase activity can also lead to low testosterone levels in some patients. In addition to low testosterone levels, the resulting elevation in estradiol may also contribute to the clinical consequences of male hypogonadism as discussed earlier. Aromatase inhibitors decrease the conversion of testosterone to estradiol, thereby increasing total testosterone levels and suppressing estradiol levels in both infertile and elderly men with borderline-low or low serum testosterone levels and can be an effective treatment option.[108,109]

Clomiphene citrate is a selective estrogen receptor modulator that has also been used in the treatment of male hypogonadism with studies suggesting an improvement in sperm production, fertility, testosterone levels, and sexual function.[110] However, clomiphene can also lead to increased estrogen levels; further study is required to determine its therapeutic potential.

SUMMARY

Decades of data support the notion that male hypogonadism is associated with not only sexual, physical, and psychological consequences but also an increase in cardiovascular risk factors and all-cause mortality. As would be expected, several small studies and meta-analyses of randomized, placebo-controlled trials have shown several benefits of testosterone replacement therapy, including decreased risk of the metabolic syndrome as well as decreased cardiovascular and all-cause mortality.

With the recent trend toward increased testosterone marketing and prescription, however, there has been a growing concern of the risk of testosterone therapy on cardiovascular events seen mostly in retrospective analyses. Unfortunately, these studies suffer from considerable limitations due to study design, inappropriate participant selection, or lack of guideline-recommended

monitoring of on-treatment testosterone levels. As with most hormonal therapies, both low and high levels may lead to adverse outcomes, confounding the interpretation of these study results. Indeed, although limited by its retrospective study design, the most recent and largest retrospective cohort study of men with testosterone deficiency found a decrease in both all-cause mortality and myocardial infarction in men who were treated with testosterone replacement and had normalization of testosterone levels on follow-up compared with untreated men and decreased all-cause mortality compared with treated men who did not normalize testosterone levels on follow-up.[94] Similarly, a well-conducted prospective study with appropriate patient selection, adequate treatment, and appropriate monitoring for dosing and safety in diabetic men found improved survival with testosterone therapy but was limited by its observational design.[84] Both of these studies are, however, limited by potential unmeasured differences in the men who were treated versus those who were not given that these studies are not randomized. Furthermore, although the largest meta-analysis of 75 randomized placebo-controlled trials did not show increased cardiovascular risk with testosterone therapy,[83] there have been no large randomized controlled trials of men with appropriately diagnosed clinical androgen deficiency on testosterone replacement with adequate monitoring and long-term follow-up data. This finding is in sharp contrast to the large randomized trials of estrogen and progesterone in women.

The authors, therefore, conclude that testosterone replacement therapy should be prescribed to hypogonadal men who have both clinical symptoms of testosterone deficiency and unequivocally low testosterone levels rather than either of these alone in accordance with a recent safety announcement from the US Food and Drug Administration.[111] As per guideline recommendations, men must have close safety monitoring, including follow-up testosterone levels that are in the midnormal range, to ensure adequate treatment and avoid the potential adverse effects of abnormally high testosterone levels. Men with cardiovascular disease or significant risk factors and concomitant hypogonadism can safely be considered for testosterone replacement therapy after discussion of the potential risks with patients. This therapy should only be undertaken if patients have true symptoms of androgen deficiency and unequivocally low testosterone levels and with close monitoring for both cardiovascular symptoms as well as on-treatment hemoglobin and testosterone levels.

The patient in the aforementioned clinical case has had years of exposure to a multitude of risk factors for coronary artery disease, and a causal effect of testosterone therapy and his incident myocardial infarction cannot be established. Furthermore, OSA can result in hormonal aberrations contributing to hypogonadism as discussed earlier; this condition should be sought and treated before initiating testosterone therapy. Treatment with testosterone therapy involves adequate monitoring, including both hematocrit as well as follow-up testosterone levels. This patient's testosterone level on testosterone therapy was 1130 ng/dL, which is well more than the midnormal range that is recommended by the Endocrine Society's clinical practice guideline.[1] This case demonstrates the potential risks and pitfalls of testosterone replacement therapy. It is likely that both low and high levels of testosterone result in adverse outcomes; this patient's suboptimal follow-up with on-treatment testosterone levels well more than the recommended treatment goal may have contributed added risk to a lifetime of cardiovascular risk exposure, the summation of which led to acute plaque rupture causing myocardial infarction.

The current data do not support the notion that testosterone therapy increases cardiovascular morbidity but certainly suggests that widespread use of testosterone supplementation without appropriate diagnosis or adequate monitoring is highly prevalent and may explain the increase in cardiovascular events seen in recent studies. All patients with cardiovascular risk factors with or without manifest cardiovascular disease should receive treatment and counseling to lower their risk of future cardiovascular events. Treatment of appropriately diagnosed hypogonadism in such patients is not contraindicated, albeit with cautious monitoring for the development of cardiovascular signs or symptoms and to ensure testosterone levels in the midnormal range and normal hematocrit levels. Given the continued discrepancy in recent trials, we should remain appropriately critical but open to the idea that testosterone replacement should be considered in men with appropriately diagnosed hypogonadism as we would any other hormone replacement therapy. In accordance with this, the authors' patient has undergone aggressive risk factor modification of his numerous cardiovascular risk factors and is currently receiving smaller doses of testosterone replacement therapy with close safety monitoring, has achieved therapeutic testosterone levels per guideline recommendations, and is maintaining cardiovascular stability with an optimal quality of life.

REFERENCES

1. Bhasin S, Cunningham GR, Hayes FJ, et al. Testosterone therapy in men with androgen deficiency syndromes: an Endocrine Society clinical practice guideline. J Clin Endocrinol Metab 2010;95(6):2536–59.
2. Baillargeon J, Urban RJ, Ottenbacher KJ, et al. Trends in androgen prescribing in the United States, 2001 to 2011. JAMA Intern Med 2013; 173(15):1465–6.
3. Gan EH, Pattman S, H S Pearce S, et al. A UK epidemic of testosterone prescribing, 2001-2010. Clin Endocrinol 2013;79(4):564–70.
4. Araujo AB, O'Donnell AB, Brambilla DJ, et al. Prevalence and incidence of androgen deficiency in middle-aged and older men: estimates from the Massachusetts Male Aging Study. J Clin Endocrinol Metab 2004;89(12):5920–6.
5. Harman SM, Metter EJ, Tobin JD, et al. Longitudinal effects of aging on serum total and free testosterone levels in healthy men. Baltimore Longitudinal Study of Aging. J Clin Endocrinol Metab 2001; 86(2):724–31.
6. Feldman HA, Longcope C, Derby CA, et al. Age trends in the level of serum testosterone and other hormones in middle-aged men: longitudinal results from the Massachusetts Male Aging Study. J Clin Endocrinol Metab 2002;87(2):589–98.
7. Wu FC, Tajar A, Pye SR, et al. Hypothalamic-pituitary-testicular axis disruptions in older men are differentially linked to age and modifiable risk factors: the European Male Aging Study. J Clin Endocrinol Metab 2008;93(7):2737–45.
8. Kaufman JM, Vermeulen A. The decline of androgen levels in elderly men and its clinical and therapeutic implications. Endocr Rev 2005; 26(6):833–76.
9. Food and Drug Administration, Center for Drug Evaluation and Research. Androgel® (testosterone) BPCA drug use review. 2009. Available at: http://www.fda.gov/downloads/AdvisoryCommittees/CommitteesMeetingMaterials/PediatricAdvisoryCommittee/UCM166697.pdf. Accessed August 29, 2014.
10. Davidson JM, Chen JJ, Crapo L, et al. Hormonal changes and sexual function in aging men. J Clin Endocrinol Metab 1983;57(1):71–7.
11. Wu FC, Tajar A, Beynon JM, et al. Identification of late-onset hypogonadism in middle-aged and elderly men. N Engl J Med 2010;363(2): 123–35.
12. Araujo AB, Esche GR, Kupelian V, et al. Prevalence of symptomatic androgen deficiency in men. J Clin Endocrinol Metab 2007;92(11):4241–7.
13. Zitzmann M, Faber S, Nieschlag E. Association of specific symptoms and metabolic risks with serum

testosterone in older men. J Clin Endocrinol Metab 2006;91(11):4335–43.

14. Riggs BL, Khosla S, Melton LJ 3rd. Sex steroids and the construction and conservation of the adult skeleton. Endocr Rev 2002;23(3):279–302.

15. van den Beld AW, de Jong FH, Grobbee DE, et al. Measures of bioavailable serum testosterone and estradiol and their relationships with muscle strength, bone density, and body composition in elderly men. J Clin Endocrinol Metab 2000;85(9): 3276–82.

16. Meier C, Nguyen TV, Handelsman DJ, et al. Endogenous sex hormones and incident fracture risk in older men: the Dubbo Osteoporosis Epidemiology Study. Arch Intern Med 2008;168(1):47–54.

17. Joshi D, van Schoor NM, de Ronde W, et al. Low free testosterone levels are associated with prevalence and incidence of depressive symptoms in older men. Clin Endocrinol 2010;72(2):232–40.

18. Shores MM, Sloan KL, Matsumoto AM, et al. Increased incidence of diagnosed depressive illness in hypogonadal older men. Arch Gen Psychiatry 2004;61(2):162–7.

19. Moffat SD, Zonderman AB, Metter EJ, et al. Longitudinal assessment of serum free testosterone concentration predicts memory performance and cognitive status in elderly men. J Clin Endocrinol Metab 2002;87(11):5001–7.

20. Haffner SM, Karhapaa P, Mykkanen L, et al. Insulin resistance, body fat distribution, and sex hormones in men. Diabetes 1994;43(2):212–9.

21. Laaksonen DE, Niskanen L, Punnonen K, et al. Testosterone and sex hormone-binding globulin predict the metabolic syndrome and diabetes in middle-aged men. Diabetes care 2004;27(5): 1036–41.

22. Oh JY, Barrett-Connor E, Wedick NM, et al. Endogenous sex hormones and the development of type 2 diabetes in older men and women: the Rancho Bernardo study. Diabetes care 2002;25(1):55–60.

23. Stellato RK, Feldman HA, Hamdy O, et al. Testosterone, sex hormone-binding globulin, and the development of type 2 diabetes in middle-aged men: prospective results from the Massachusetts Male Aging Study. Diabetes care 2000;23(4): 490–4.

24. Ding EL, Song Y, Malik VS, et al. Sex differences of endogenous sex hormones and risk of type 2 diabetes: a systematic review and meta-analysis. JAMA 2006;295(11):1288–99.

25. Muller M, Grobbee DE, den Tonkelaar I, et al. Endogenous sex hormones and metabolic syndrome in aging men. J Clin Endocrinol Metab 2005;90(5):2618–23.

26. Khaw KT, Barrett-Connor E. Lower endogenous androgens predict central adiposity in men. Ann Epidemiol 1992;2(5):675–82.

27. Tchernof A, Labrie F, Belanger A, et al. Relationships between endogenous steroid hormone, sex hormone-binding globulin and lipoprotein levels in men: contribution of visceral obesity, insulin levels and other metabolic variables. Atherosclerosis 1997;133(2):235–44.

28. Haring R, Baumeister SE, Volzke H, et al. Prospective association of low total testosterone concentrations with an adverse lipid profile and increased incident dyslipidemia. Eur J Cardiovasc Prev Rehabil 2011;18(1):86–96.

29. Zmuda JM, Cauley JA, Kriska A, et al. Longitudinal relation between endogenous testosterone and cardiovascular disease risk factors in middle-aged men. A 13-year follow-up of former Multiple Risk Factor Intervention Trial participants. Am J Epidemiol 1997;146(8):609–17.

30. Makinen JI, Perheentupa A, Irjala K, et al. Endogenous testosterone and serum lipids in middle-aged men. Atherosclerosis 2008;197(2):688–93.

31. Kupelian V, Page ST, Araujo AB, et al. Low sex hormone-binding globulin, total testosterone, and symptomatic androgen deficiency are associated with development of the metabolic syndrome in nonobese men. J Clin Endocrinol Metab 2006; 91(3):843–50.

32. Fukui M, Kitagawa Y, Nakamura N, et al. Association between serum testosterone concentration and carotid atherosclerosis in men with type 2 diabetes. Diabetes care 2003; 26(6):1869–73.

33. Muller M, van den Beld AW, Bots ML, et al. Endogenous sex hormones and progression of carotid atherosclerosis in elderly men. Circulation 2004; 109(17):2074–9.

34. Svartberg J, von Muhlen D, Mathiesen E, et al. Low testosterone levels are associated with carotid atherosclerosis in men. J Intern Med 2006;259(6): 576–82.

35. Tivesten A, Mellstrom D, Jutberger H, et al. Low serum testosterone and high serum estradiol associate with lower extremity peripheral arterial disease in elderly men. The MrOS Study in Sweden. J Am Coll Cardiol 2007;50(11):1070–6.

36. Kaplan SA, Johnson-Levonas AO, Lin J, et al. Elevated high sensitivity C-reactive protein levels in aging men with low testosterone. Aging Male 2010;13(2):108–12.

37. Tivesten A, Vandenput L, Labrie F, et al. Low serum testosterone and estradiol predict mortality in elderly men. J Clin Endocrinol Metab 2009;94(7): 2482–8.

38. Laughlin GA, Barrett-Connor E, Bergstrom J. Low serum testosterone and mortality in older men. J Clin Endocrinol Metab 2008;93(1):68–75.

39. Haring R, Volzke H, Steveling A, et al. Low serum testosterone levels are associated with increased

risk of mortality in a population-based cohort of men aged 20-79. Eur Heart J 2010;31(12):1494–501.

40. Shores MM, Matsumoto AM, Sloan KL, et al. Low serum testosterone and mortality in male veterans. Arch Intern Med 2006;166(15):1660–5.

41. Khaw KT, Dowsett M, Folkerd E, et al. Endogenous testosterone and mortality due to all causes, cardiovascular disease, and cancer in men: European prospective investigation into cancer in Norfolk (EPIC-Norfolk) Prospective Population Study. Circulation 2007;116(23):2694–701.

42. Hyde Z, Norman PE, Flicker L, et al. Low free testosterone predicts mortality from cardiovascular disease but not other causes: the Health in Men Study. J Clin Endocrinol Metab 2012;97(1): 179–89.

43. Ohlsson C, Barrett-Connor E, Bhasin S, et al. High serum testosterone is associated with reduced risk of cardiovascular events in elderly men. The MrOS (Osteoporotic Fractures in Men) study in Sweden. J Am Coll Cardiol 2011;58(16):1674–81.

44. Corona G, Rastrelli G, Monami M, et al. Hypogonadism as a risk factor for cardiovascular mortality in men: a meta-analytic study. Eur J Endocrinol 2011;165(5):687–701.

45. Araujo AB, Dixon JM, Suarez EA, et al. Clinical review: endogenous testosterone and mortality in men: a systematic review and meta-analysis. J Clin Endocrinol Metab 2011;96(10):3007–19.

46. Malkin CJ, Pugh PJ, Morris PD, et al. Low serum testosterone and increased mortality in men with coronary heart disease. Heart 2010;96(22):1821–5.

47. Smith GD, Ben-Shlomo Y, Beswick A, et al. Cortisol, testosterone, and coronary heart disease: prospective evidence from the Caerphilly study. Circulation 2005;112(3):332–40.

48. Araujo AB, Kupelian V, Page ST, et al. Sex steroids and all-cause and cause-specific mortality in men. Arch Intern Med 2007;167(12):1252–60.

49. Ruige JB, Mahmoud AM, De Bacquer D, et al. Endogenous testosterone and cardiovascular disease in healthy men: a meta-analysis. Heart 2011; 97(11):870–5.

50. Keating NL, O'Malley AJ, Smith MR. Diabetes and cardiovascular disease during androgen deprivation therapy for prostate cancer. J Clin Oncol 2006;24(27):4448–56.

51. Levine GN, D'Amico AV, Berger P, et al. Androgen-deprivation therapy in prostate cancer and cardiovascular risk: a science advisory from the American Heart Association, American Cancer Society, and American Urological Association: endorsed by the American Society for Radiation Oncology. Circulation 2010;121(6):833–40.

52. Bolona ER, Uraga MV, Haddad RM, et al. Testosterone use in men with sexual dysfunction: a systematic review and meta-analysis of randomized placebo-controlled trials. Mayo Clin Proc 2007; 82(1):20–8.

53. Allan CA, Forbes EA, Strauss BJ, et al. Testosterone therapy increases sexual desire in ageing men with low-normal testosterone levels and symptoms of androgen deficiency. Int J Impot Res 2008; 20(4):396–401.

54. Wang C, Swerdloff RS, Iranmanesh A, et al. Transdermal testosterone gel improves sexual function, mood, muscle strength, and body composition parameters in hypogonadal men. J Clin Endocrinol Metab 2000;85(8):2839–53.

55. Katznelson L, Finkelstein JS, Schoenfeld DA, et al. Increase in bone density and lean body mass during testosterone administration in men with acquired hypogonadism. J Clin Endocrinol Metab 1996;81(12):4358–65.

56. Bhasin S, Storer TW, Berman N, et al. Testosterone replacement increases fat-free mass and muscle size in hypogonadal men. J Clin Endocrinol Metab 1997;82(2):407–13.

57. Behre HM, Kliesch S, Leifke E, et al. Long-term effect of testosterone therapy on bone mineral density in hypogonadal men. J Clin Endocrinol Metab 1997;82(8):2386–90.

58. Snyder PJ, Peachey H, Berlin JA, et al. Effects of testosterone replacement in hypogonadal men. J Clin Endocrinol Metab 2000;85(8):2670–7.

59. Steidle C, Schwartz S, Jacoby K, et al. AA2500 testosterone gel normalizes androgen levels in aging males with improvements in body composition and sexual function. J Clin Endocrinol Metab 2003;88(6):2673–81.

60. Wang C, Cunningham G, Dobs A, et al. Long-term testosterone gel (AndroGel) treatment maintains beneficial effects on sexual function and mood, lean and fat mass, and bone mineral density in hypogonadal men. J Clin Endocrinol Metab 2004; 89(5):2085–98.

61. Aminorroaya A, Kelleher S, Conway AJ, et al. Adequacy of androgen replacement influences bone density response to testosterone in androgen-deficient men. Eur J Endocrinol 2005; 152(6):881–6.

62. Srinivas-Shankar U, Roberts SA, Connolly MJ, et al. Effects of testosterone on muscle strength, physical function, body composition, and quality of life in intermediate-frail and frail elderly men: a randomized, double-blind, placebo-controlled study. J Clin Endocrinol Metab 2010;95(2):639–50.

63. Zarrouf FA, Artz S, Griffith J, et al. Testosterone and depression: systematic review and meta-analysis. J Psychiatr Pract 2009;15(4):289–305.

64. Kapoor D, Goodwin E, Channer KS, et al. Testosterone replacement therapy improves insulin resistance, glycaemic control, visceral adiposity and hypercholesterolaemia in hypogonadal men

with type 2 diabetes. Eur J Endocrinol 2006; 154(6):899–906.

65. Jones TH, Arver S, Behre HM, et al. Testosterone replacement in hypogonadal men with type 2 diabetes and/or metabolic syndrome (the TIMES2 study). Diabetes care 2011;34(4):828–37.

66. Heufelder AE, Saad F, Bunck MC, et al. Fifty-two-week treatment with diet and exercise plus transdermal testosterone reverses the metabolic syndrome and improves glycemic control in men with newly diagnosed type 2 diabetes and subnormal plasma testosterone. J Androl 2009; 30(6):726–33.

67. Kalinchenko SY, Tishova YA, Mskhalaya GJ, et al. Effects of testosterone supplementation on markers of the metabolic syndrome and inflammation in hypogonadal men with the metabolic syndrome: the double-blinded placebo-controlled Moscow study. Clin Endocrinol 2010; 73(5):602–12.

68. Corona G, Monami M, Rastrelli G, et al. Testosterone and metabolic syndrome: a meta-analysis study. J Sex Med 2011;8(1):272–83.

69. English KM, Steeds RP, Jones TH, et al. Low-dose transdermal testosterone therapy improves angina threshold in men with chronic stable angina: a randomized, double-blind, placebo-controlled study. Circulation 2000;102(16):1906–11.

70. Mathur A, Malkin C, Saeed B, et al. Long-term benefits of testosterone replacement therapy on angina threshold and atheroma in men. Eur J Endocrinol 2009;161(3):443–9.

71. Malkin CJ, Pugh PJ, West JN, et al. Testosterone therapy in men with moderate severity heart failure: a double-blind randomized placebo controlled trial. Eur Heart J 2006;27(1):57–64.

72. Caminiti G, Volterrani M, Iellamo F, et al. Effect of long-acting testosterone treatment on functional exercise capacity, skeletal muscle performance, insulin resistance, and baroreflex sensitivity in elderly patients with chronic heart failure a double-blind, placebo-controlled, randomized study. J Am Coll Cardiol 2009;54(10):919–27.

73. Basaria S, Harman SM, Travison TG, et al. Effects of testosterone administration for 3 years on subclinical atherosclerosis progression in older men with low or low-normal testosterone levels: a randomized clinical trial. JAMA 2015; 314(6):570–81.

74. Salameh WA, Redor-Goldman MM, Clarke NJ, et al. Validation of a total testosterone assay using high-turbulence liquid chromatography tandem mass spectrometry: total and free testosterone reference ranges. Steroids 2010;75(2):169–75.

75. Endocrine Society. The risk of cardiovascular events in men receiving testosterone therapy. An Endocrine Society statement. 2014. Available at:

https://www.endocrine.org/~/media/endosociety/ Files/Advocacy%20and%20Outreach/Position% 20Statements/Other%20Statements/The%20Risk% 20of%20Cardiovascular%20Events%20in%20Men% 20Receiving%20Testosterone%20Therapy.pdf. Accessed August 29, 2014.

76. Basaria S, Coviello AD, Travison TG, et al. Adverse events associated with testosterone administration. N Engl J Med 2010;363(2):109–22.

77. Basaria S, Davda MN, Travison TG, et al. Risk factors associated with cardiovascular events during testosterone administration in older men with mobility limitation. J Gerontol A Biol Sci Med Sci 2013;68(2):153–60.

78. Xu L, Freeman G, Cowling BJ, et al. Testosterone therapy and cardiovascular events among men: a systematic review and meta-analysis of placebo-controlled randomized trials. BMC Med 2013;11:108.

79. Haddad RM, Kennedy CC, Caples SM, et al. Testosterone and cardiovascular risk in men: a systematic review and meta-analysis of randomized placebo-controlled trials. Mayo Clin Proc 2007; 82(1):29–39.

80. Carson CC 3rd, Rosano G. Exogenous testosterone, cardiovascular events, and cardiovascular risk factors in elderly men: a review of trial data. J Sex Med 2012;9(1):54–67.

81. Calof OM, Singh AB, Lee ML, et al. Adverse events associated with testosterone replacement in middle-aged and older men: a meta-analysis of randomized, placebo-controlled trials. J Gerontol A Biol Sci Med Sci 2005;60(11):1451–7.

82. Fernandez-Balsells MM, Murad MH, Lane M, et al. Clinical review 1: adverse effects of testosterone therapy in adult men: a systematic review and meta-analysis. J Clin Endocrinol Metab 2010; 95(6):2560–75.

83. Corona G, Maseroli E, Rastrelli G, et al. Cardiovascular risk associated with testosterone-boosting medications: a systematic review and meta-analysis. Expert Opin Drug Saf 2014;13(10):1327–51.

84. Muraleedharan V, Marsh H, Kapoor D, et al. Testosterone deficiency is associated with increased risk of mortality and testosterone replacement improves survival in men with type 2 diabetes. Eur J Endocrinol 2013;169(6):725–33.

85. Vigen R, O'Donnell CI, Baron AE, et al. Association of testosterone therapy with mortality, myocardial infarction, and stroke in men with low testosterone levels. JAMA 2013;310(17):1829–36.

86. Morgentaler A, Traish A, Kacker R. Deaths and cardiovascular events in men receiving testosterone. JAMA 2014;311(9):961–2.

87. Jones TH, Channer KS. Deaths and cardiovascular events in men receiving testosterone. JAMA 2014; 311(9):962–3.

88. Katz J, Nadelberg R. Deaths and cardiovascular events in men receiving testosterone. JAMA 2014;311(9):963.

89. Riche DM, Baker WL, Koch CA. Deaths and cardiovascular events in men receiving testosterone. JAMA 2014;311(9):963–4.

90. Dhindsa S, Batra M, Dandona P. Deaths and cardiovascular events in men receiving testosterone. JAMA 2014;311(9):964.

91. Finkle WD, Greenland S, Ridgeway GK, et al. Increased risk of non-fatal myocardial infarction following testosterone therapy prescription in men. PLoS One 2014;9(1):e85805.

92. Layton JB, Meier CR, Sharpless JL, et al. Comparative safety of testosterone dosage forms. JAMA Intern Med 2015;175(7):1187–96.

93. Shores MM, Smith NL, Forsberg CW, et al. Testosterone treatment and mortality in men with low testosterone levels. J Clin Endocrinol Metab 2012; 97(6):2050–8.

94. Sharma R, Oni OA, Gupta K, et al. Normalization of testosterone level is associated with reduced incidence of myocardial infarction and mortality in men. Eur Heart J 2015;36(40):2706–15.

95. McCrohon JA, Jessup W, Handelsman DJ, et al. Androgen exposure increases human monocyte adhesion to vascular endothelium and endothelial cell expression of vascular cell adhesion molecule-1. Circulation 1999;99(17):2317–22.

96. Death AK, McGrath KC, Sader MA, et al. Dihydrotestosterone promotes vascular cell adhesion molecule-1 expression in male human endothelial cells via a nuclear factor-kappaB-dependent pathway. Endocrinology 2004;145(4):1889–97.

97. Shores MM, Biggs ML, Arnold AM, et al. Testosterone, dihydrotestosterone, and incident cardiovascular disease and mortality in the cardiovascular health study. J Clin Endocrinol Metab 2014;99(6):2061–8.

98. Ajayi AA, Mathur R, Halushka PV. Testosterone increases human platelet thromboxane A2 receptor density and aggregation responses. Circulation 1995;91(11):2742–7.

99. Marchioli R, Finazzi G, Specchia G, et al. Cardiovascular events and intensity of treatment in polycythemia vera. N Engl J Med 2013;368(1): 22–33.

100. Hoyos CM, Killick R, Yee BJ, et al. Effects of testosterone therapy on sleep and breathing in obese men with severe obstructive sleep apnoea: a randomized placebo-controlled trial. Clin Endocrinol 2012;77(4):599–607.

101. Swerdloff RS, Wang C, Cunningham G, et al. Long-term pharmacokinetics of transdermal testosterone gel in hypogonadal men. J Clin Endocrinol Metab 2000;85(12):4500–10.

102. Lakshman KM, Kaplan B, Travison TG, et al. The effects of injected testosterone dose and age on the conversion of testosterone to estradiol and dihydrotestosterone in young and older men. J Clin Endocrinol Metab 2010;95(8):3955–64.

103. Phillips GB, Pinkernell BH, Jing TY. The association of hyperestrogenemia with coronary thrombosis in men. Arterioscler Thromb Vasc Biol 1996;16(11):1383–7.

104. Abbott RD, Launer LJ, Rodriguez BL, et al. Serum estradiol and risk of stroke in elderly men. Neurology 2007;68(8):563–8.

105. The Coronary Drug Project. Initial findings leading to modifications of its research protocol. JAMA 1970;214(7):1303–13.

106. Shamloul R, Ghanem H. Erectile dysfunction. Lancet 2013;381(9861):153–65.

107. Miner M, Nehra A, Jackson G, et al. All men with vasculogenic erectile dysfunction require a cardiovascular workup. Am J Med 2014;127(3): 174–82.

108. Schlegel PN. Aromatase inhibitors for male infertility. Fertil Steril 2012;98(6):1359–62.

109. Leder BZ, Rohrer JL, Rubin SD, et al. Effects of aromatase inhibition in elderly men with low or borderline-low serum testosterone levels. J Clin Endocrinol Metab 2004;89(3):1174–80.

110. Kaminetsky J, Hemani ML. Clomiphene citrate and enclomiphene for the treatment of hypogonadal androgen deficiency. Expert Opin Investig Drugs 2009;18(12):1947–55.

111. Food and Drug Administration. FDA drug safety communication: FDA evaluating risk of stroke, heart attack and death with FDA-approved testosterone products. 2014.

Trends in Testosterone Prescription and Public Health Concerns

 CrossMark

Joseph Scott Gabrielsen, MD, PhD[a,1], Bobby B. Najari, MD[b,1],
Joseph P. Alukal, MD[c], Michael L. Eisenberg, MD[d,*]

KEYWORDS

- Testosterone supplementation therapy • Hypogonadism • Testosterone replacement therapy
- Late-onset hypogonadism

KEY POINTS

- Testosterone supplementation therapy has become increasingly popular since the turn of the century.
- In the U.S., most testosterone prescriptions are written by primary care providers, endocrinologists, or urologists.
- Due to conflicting results regarding the efficacy and safety of testosterone supplementation, the US Food and Drug Administration has asked manufacturers to clarify the labeling of these products and requested further research into the long term use of testosterone products.
- Results from these studies will help define the appropriate population for testosterone supplementation therapy going forward. It is hoped that these data combined with physician and public education will minimize inappropriate prescribing and allow those likely to benefit from testosterone supplementation therapy to receive it.

"It is important not to conclude that every old man who is tired is suffering from the male climacteric. This diagnosis should be made only after the most careful search has been carried out to discover some other cause for the symptoms."[1] This statement is from an article entitled Uses and Abuses of the Male Sex Hormone published in *The Journal of the American Medical Association* in 1946, when age-related hypogonadism was referred to as *climacteric*. The struggle to define what is appropriate use of testosterone supplementation therapy (TST) and what constitutes misuse of these drugs has been present since the hormone was first synthesized in 1935.[2]

The intensity of public scrutiny has increased with the approval and marketing of various testosterone formulations since the turn of the century. In 2002, recognizing the public interest in testosterone products, the National Institute of Aging and the National Cancer Institute requested the Institute of Medicine conduct an assessment of clinical research on TST. The study concluded that uncertainties remain regarding the use of TST in older men.[3] Further developments in both the popularity and risk profile of these medications

[a] Department of Urology, Massachusetts General Hospital, 55 Fruit Street, Boston, MA 02114, USA; [b] Department of Urology, Weill Cornell Medical College, James Buchanan Brady Foundation, 525 East 68th Street, Starr 9, New York, NY 10065, USA; [c] Departments of Urology and Obstetrics/Gynecology, New York University, 150 East 32nd Street, 2nd Floor, New York, NY 10016, USA; [d] Departments of Urology and Obstetrics and Gynecology, Stanford University School of Medicine, 300 Pasteur Drive, Stanford, CA 94305-5118, USA
[1] Co-first authors.
* Corresponding author.
E-mail address: eisenberg@stanford.edu

Urol Clin N Am 43 (2016) 261–271
http://dx.doi.org/10.1016/j.ucl.2016.01.010

have led to increasing public health concerns in recent years.

TRENDS IN THE PRESCRIPTION OF TESTOSTERONE

The continued research and development of a diverse range of testosterone formulations will continue to benefit men with hypogonadism. Much of the concern about the use of TST, however, has arisen because of the rapidly increasing number of men using TST in the United States (**Table 1**) and worldwide. Many of these men are prescribed testosterone for age-related decreases in testosterone (subsequently referred to as *late-onset hypogonadism* [LOH]) rather than classic androgen deficiency caused by pathologic conditions such as Klinefelter's syndrome, orchiectomy, and chemotherapy. The trend of increasing use of TST has been documented in a variety of ways ranging from commercial insurance claims data to integrated health care systems.

Commercial Insurance Claims Data

Layton and colleagues[4] used a commercial health insurance database, MarketScan Commercial Claims and Encounters, to evaluate trends in testosterone initiation in the United States from 2000 to 2011. The authors evaluated 410,000 men older than 18 years who initiated testosterone therapy each year. They calculated the population rates of testosterone initiation by using person-years of eligibility as the denominator (calculated by summing the continuously enrolled person-time for men in each year). The annual rate of testosterone initiation increased from 20.2 per 10,000 person-years in 2000 to 75.7 per 10,000 person-years in 2011—a nearly 4-fold increase—with an accelerating rate after 2008. Most men initiating testosterone therapy were relatively young (74% were between the ages of 40 and 64); however, commercial health insurance databases are limited by undersampling of men older than 65 who use Medicare as their primary source of health care coverage.

Baillargeon and colleagues[5] used data from Clinformatics DataMart, one of the largest commercial health insurance populations, to examine testosterone-prescribing practice patterns from the years 2001 to 2011. The authors restricted the study to men age 40 years and older to focus on the issue of testosterone use in men with LOH. The database included more than 10 million men in this age group, with at least 1 million men covered by insurance every year of the decade studied. They found that testosterone use increased 3-fold between 2001 and 2011. In 2001, 0.81% of men older than 40 years were using TST compared with 2.91% in 2011. Use of topical gel formulations of testosterone had the largest increase with a 5-fold increase during the decade. Again, one limitation of this report is its reliance on commercial health insurance, which undersamples men older than 65 years.

Pharmacy Sales

Using data obtained from IMS Consulting, the 2002 Institute of Medicine study reported that although sales of testosterone products were steady at approximately $18 million per year until 1988, the annual sales of these projects was $400 million by 2002.[6] The number of testosterone prescriptions written increased from 648,000 in 1999 to 1.75 million in 2002, a 170% increase.[3] The first gel preparation of testosterone was approved for use in the United States in 2000.

The US Food and Drug Administration (FDA) held a joint meeting between the Bone, Reproductive, and Urologic Drugs Advisory Committee and the Drug Safety and Risk Management Advisory Committee on September 17, 2014. During the meeting, Mohamed A. Mohamoud from the FDA's Office of Surveillance and Epidemiology presented recent prescription sales data using the Symphony Healthcare Solutions Anonymous Patient Longitudinal Database.[7] This database captured unique patients filling a prescription for testosterone at outpatient pharmacies throughout the nation. National projections from these data estimated that the number of men filling

Table 1
Percentage increase in the use of TST in the United States

Study	Database Type	Population	Number	Years Studied	% Increase
Baillargeon et al,[5] 2013	Commercial insurance	>40 y	10,739,815	2001–2011	359
Layton et al,[4] 2014	Commercial insurance	>18 y	410,019	2000–2010	374
Jasuja et al,[8] 2015	Veteran Affairs	>20 y	111,631	2009–2012	78
Nguyen et al,[7] 2015	Outpatient pharmacy	All ages	7,246,013	2010–2013	183

testosterone prescriptions increased from 1.2 million in 2010 to 2.2 million in 2013, a near doubling in just 4 years.

Veterans Administration Health Care System Data

The Veterans Administration (VA) Health Care System is the largest integrated health care system in United States and allows for analysis of practice patterns using medical records, laboratory tests, and prescription data. Jasuja and colleagues[8] evaluated the testosterone-prescribing practices in the VA Health Care System from fiscal years 2009 to 2012. Evaluating records from more than 6 million men who received at least 1 outpatient medication from a participating pharmacy, they found that 1.7% of the men received a new prescription for testosterone during the period. The annual number of men with new testosterone prescriptions increased from 20,437 in 2009 to 36,394 in 2012, a 78% increase over 4 years. In keeping with other studies in which age at the time of testosterone initiation was evaluated, 81.9% of men starting treatment were older than 49 years.

International Trends

In one of the earliest reports of increased testosterone prescribing around world, Handelsman[9] used the Australian Pharmaceutical Benefits Scheme (PBS) to evaluate trends in testosterone prescribing in Australia from 1991 to 2001. The PBS provides coverage for medically necessary medications and represents 80% of prescriptions written in Australia. Overall there was an increase in annual testosterone prescriptions from 14,000 in 1991 to 26,000 in 2001. The author found that regulatory changes affected prescribing trends. The number of testosterone prescriptions doubled from approximately 14,000 prescriptions written in 1991 to 32,000 in 1994. Beginning in 1994, PBS required telephone authorization for testosterone prescriptions, which resulted in a decline in testosterone prescriptions to 22,000 in 1996; however, a steady increase in prescriptions followed with annual prescriptions peaking at 31,000 by 1999. In 2000, PBS implemented further restrictions requiring conformation to Endocrine Society of Australia consensus guidelines, resulting in a decrease to 26,000 prescriptions in 2001. This study provides insight into how regulatory oversight of testosterone products can influence physician prescribing habits.

Handelsman[10] also used a pharmaceutical sales database to write a brief report on global sales of testosterone products from 2000 to 2011. He converted testosterone sales data from 41 countries

into number of monthly doses sold per year. He found that global testosterone sales increased from $150 million in 2000 to $1.8 billion in 2011, a 12-fold increase. The slope of increase was increasingly steep during the latter part of the decade. These trends were seen in all regions of the world and in 37 of the 41 countries examined. Although sales data are likely proportional to the number of men using these products, patient-level data were lacking.

Layton and colleagues[4] used the Clinical Practice Research Datalink database, a registry of health record information from general practitioners, to evaluate trends of TST in the United Kingdom from 2000 to 2010. A total of 6833 men initiated treatment during this period. The TST initiation rate increased from 3.4 per 10,000 person-years in 2000 to 4.5 per 10,000 patient-years in 2010, which was much lower than that reported in the United States. Most (83.4%) of these men were older than 39 years. This study may have underestimated the number of men initiating TST; however, prescribing data from specialists were not included in the database.

PREFERENCES IN PRESCRIBED TESTOSTERONE FORMULATIONS

Testosterone is available as short- and long-acting injectables, transdermals (ie, gels and patches), pellets, and oral formulations, although availability varies by country. Details regarding specific testosterone preparations, their uses and limitations have been detailed elsewhere in this issue (See Khera M: Testosterone therapies, in this issue).

The worldwide increase in testosterone sales has largely been attributed to the increasing use of topical formulations.[10] According to FDA data, an estimated 59,000 kg of testosterone products were sold in the United States between 2009 and 2013, with 71% of those products being testosterone gels.[11] In Ontario, Canada, expenditures on topical preparations increased 464% between 2007 and 2012.[12] The increase in testosterone prescribing seems to be blunted where formulary restrictions limit coverage of topical formulations, such as the Veterans Administration Health Care System in the United States.[13]

This increase in prescribing reflects prescriber preferences. Among specialists prescribing TST, 62% reported a preference for testosterone gel when initiating treatment; 55% preferred gels for long-term treatment.[14] Analysis of the geographic distribution of respondents found that testosterone gels were the preferred formulation among North American clinicians, whereas long-lasting injections were preferred among non–North American clinicians.[14] This finding is somewhat misleading, as the long-lasting injection was only recently approved by the FDA for use in the United States and, therefore, would not have been available to those prescribers at the time of the study. Thus, formulation preferences are likely to evolve as practitioners become more familiar with newer options. A separate survey limited to European testosterone prescribers (45% general practitioners, 31% urologists, and 24% endocrinologists) found that 26% preferred long-acting intramuscular injections, 24% gels, 21% matrix transdermal device, 15% short-acting injections, and 13% oral formulations.[15]

TESTOSTERONE PRESCRIBER DEMOGRAPHICS

Although there is variation based on the population sampled, most testosterone prescribers in the United States and Canada are primary care providers. In a large US health care system, 73% of TST prescribers were found to be primary care providers, 16% were endocrinologists, and 5% were urologists.[16] Analysis of the Truven Marketscan Database found 59% of prescribers were primary care providers and 18% were urologists.[17] Similarly, the FDA reported that 60% of US prescribers were primary care providers.[7] Interestingly, a survey of men with hypogonadism already diagnosed in the United States found they were actively seeking treatment most commonly from a urologist (30.5%) followed by a general practitioner (28%),[18] but this may not reflect which provider initiated TST. In Canada, family physicians initiated 66% to 78% of new prescriptions.[12,19]

Although multiple studies have evaluated the distribution of providers prescribing TST, only one study evaluated changes in providers' prescribing patterns with time. A worldwide survey of members of the major endocrine and andrology societies (91% of respondents were endocrinologists) found wide variation in practice patterns.[14] When queried about their inclination to treat borderline hypogonadal men with nonspecific symptoms, 46% reported being less inclined to do so now than they were 5 years ago, whereas 30% reported no change. This trend was stronger among participants from North America and Oceania than in other parts of the world.[14]

A survey of TST prescribers in Europe found that 74% considered that both symptoms and low testosterone levels were required for the diagnosis of testosterone deficiency syndrome in men.[15] Although data regarding reasons for prescribing TST have not been published, a survey of 353 frequent TST prescribers from 6 large, non-US countries evaluated reasons for physicians not prescribing TST. Physicians reported initiating TST in approximately two-thirds of hypogonadal patients. Prostate cancer concerns were the primary reasons for not initiating TST.[20] Of note, although 68% of physicians associated TST with side effects, 32% expressed a belief that there were no side effects.[20]

TESTOSTERONE USER DEMOGRAPHICS

FDA data indicate that 97% of testosterone prescriptions in the United States were to men and 3% to women in 2013.[11] Men younger than 40 years accounted for 13% of prescriptions, whereas men between 40 and 60 years accounted for 70%.[11] Similar data have been reported by Malik and colleagues,[16] who found that 27% of the new testosterone prescriptions in the United States in 2012 were to men younger than 40 years and 30% to men younger than 50 years. According to FDA data, the 40- to 60-year age group saw the largest relative increase in prescribing between 2010 and 2013.[11] Canup and colleagues[21] reported that testosterone prescriptions increased an average of 33% per year between 2007 and 2011 among the 18- to 44-year-old men in the United States military.[21]

Similar results were reported in Canada. Analysis of prescriptions in Winnipeg, Canada, found 14% of prescriptions were to men less than 40 years and 58% to men 40 to 60 years.[19]

Reasons for patient initiation of TST are not well reported in the literature; however, data suggest that both specific and nonspecific symptoms of testosterone deficiency are the likely cause. For example, among 127 men with symptomatic testosterone deficiency (defined as a total serum testosterone level <300 ng/dL or free testosterone level <1.5 ng/dL), most patients complained of erectile dysfunction and low libido (65%), whereas fatigue was reported in 21% and an altered sense of well-being in 19%.[22] Another study of US men with hypogonadism found that the most common symptoms driving them to seek treatment were erectile dysfunction (66%), loss of energy/increased tiredness (59%), and decreased sex drive (58%).[18]

Men who undergo testosterone testing and are initiated on testosterone frequently have comorbid conditions such as obesity, diabetes, and hypertension,[12] and poor health has been associated with steeper declines in testosterone levels with aging.[23] Many studies report age-related declines in testosterone.[23–25] Interestingly, the MAILES

(Men Androgens Inflammation Lifestyle Environment and Stress) study reported that serum testosterone levels were essentially unchanged over the course of 5 years in healthy men, suggesting that the age-related decline in testosterone levels may be caused by changes in comorbid conditions rather than aging itself.[26]

Investigators also reported secular declines in testosterone levels in men. Data from the Massachusetts Male Aging Study reported declines in age-adjusted testosterone levels in men based on decade of recruitment from the 1980s to the 2000s suggesting that men at risk for hypogonadism may be increasing.[25]

PRACTICE PATTERNS INCONSISTENT WITH MEDICAL ORGANIZATION GUIDELINES

By 2005, multiple medical societies issued guidelines for the diagnosis and management of hypogonadism, including the Endocrine Society, American Society of Andrology, International Society of Andrology, European Society of Andrology, and European Association of Urology.[27–30] Although there is some variation in their recommendations, one consistent message is that TST should only be prescribed to symptomatic men in whom low serum testosterone is document on 2 appropriately obtained laboratory tests. Much of the public health concern surrounding TST is that the increase in testosterone use does not reflect best practices (**Table 2**).

In the initial report by Baillargeon and colleagues,[5] approximately 25% of men prescribed TST did not have a documented serum testosterone level during the preceding 12 months. In 2015, Baillargeon and colleagues[31] updated their analysis of the same population and reported that only 18% of men had the recommended 2 serum testosterone tests before initiation of treatment. Among the men who did have testosterone testing before treatment, 20% had serum

testosterone levels within the normal range. Men who saw either an endocrinologist or urologist were more likely to have appropriate testing before therapy; however, those who saw a urologist were more likely to initiate TST despite a normal testosterone value.

Layton and colleagues[4] also compared testosterone laboratory testing and TST initiation trends in the United States and the United Kingdom between 2000 and 2011. They identified 1.1 million men in the United States and 66,140 men in the United Kingdom who had a new laboratory test for testosterone during that period. Although the rate of testosterone testing increased in both countries, the slope of increase was much steeper in the United States, especially after 2008. Increased testing in the United Kingdom was associated with an increase the percentage of test results falling below the normal range (18.9% in 2000%–26.7% in 2011). In the United States, however, the opposite was true—the proportion of normal results increased from 64.5% to 73.2% between 2007 and 2011. These data suggest that increased testing in the United States, presumably because of increased awareness of the symptoms of hypogonadism, was not accompanied by increased accuracy in physician suspicion for the condition. This finding is supported by their findings that fatigue was more frequently cited as the indication for testosterone testing in the United States compared with the United Kingdom.

Like other studies, the most concerning finding from this study was inadequate laboratory testing before initiation of TST. In the United States, 90% of men starting TST did not have 2 testosterone levels and 40% had no testosterone levels measured during the preceding 6 months. Likewise, in the United Kingdom, 87% and 54% did not have 2 or any tests, respectively. Whereas men in the United Kingdom were more likely to start TST without prior testing, men in the United

Table 2
Percentage of men undergoing appropriate pretreatment evaluation

Study	Database Type	Population	Number	Number of Pretreatment Tests (%)		
				0	1	2
Layton et al,[4] 2014	Commercial insurance	>18 y	410,029	40	50	10
Muram et al,[32] 2015	Commercial insurance	>18 y	63,534	29	31	40
Jasuja et al,[8] 2015	Veteran Affairs	>20 y	111,631	16.5	83.5	
Baillargeon et al,[31] 2015	Commercial insurance	>40 y	61,474	24.6	57.4	18

States were more likely to start TST despite normal serum testosterone levels (9% vs 1%). Although this study did not capture testosterone testing ordered more than 6 months before TST initiation or tests paid for out of pocket, these data suggest that many practitioners are not evaluating and treating patients for hypogonadism in accordance with guidelines.

Muram and colleagues[32] published an industry-sponsored study using another commercial health insurance database, the Truven Health Market-scan Commercial and Medicare Supplemental Insurance Databases, to evaluate hormone testing for hypogonadism from 2010 to 2012. This cohort consisted of 63,000 men 18 years and older who initiated TST and were continuously insured at least 12 months before and 6 months after initiation. They reported that although 40% had at least 2 testosterone levels measured before initiation, 29% were treated without any laboratory assessment. Furthermore, only 12% of men had any assessment of their pituitary function through measurement of gonadotropins. Men were more likely to have had testosterone assessed before initiating testosterone therapy if they had seen an endocrinologist (80%) compared with urologists (70%) or primary care providers (71%). Likewise, men were more likely to have a pituitary function assessment before testosterone therapy if they had seen an endocrinologist (45%) as opposed to urologists (15%) or primary care providers (10%).

Jasuja and colleagues[8] also found inappropriate initiation of TST within the VA Health Care System. The authors found that only 5.4% of men with a diagnosis of hypogonadism had 2 or more low testosterone levels obtained in the morning, a practice consistent with clinical guidelines. Only 18.3% had 2 low testosterone levels (drawn at any time of the day). The authors found that 16.5% of men did not have any testosterone measurements assessed before initiation of TST.

The integrated nature of the VA Health Care System also allowed Jasuja and colleagues[8] to ascertain how many men were prescribed testosterone despite contraindications to such therapy. Relative contraindications such as obstructive sleep apnea, hematocrit greater than 50%, and PSA level greater than 4.0 ng/dL were present in 12.9% of men. Absolute contraindications of prostate cancer and breast cancer were present in 1.4% of men. The authors' most striking finding was that only 3.1% of men filling testosterone prescriptions in the VA Health Care System had care consistent with published guidelines.

Additionally, TST in reproductive-age men goes against society recommendations, especially if fertility impacts are not discussed with the patient.

Although many of the side effects of TST may be debated, there is little debate regarding the impact of testosterone on fertility. Testosterone is essential for spermatogenesis; however, exogenous testosterone supplementation effectively induces oligospermia and azoospermia in healthy men.[33,34] Impairment of spermatogenesis occurs through inhibition of the hypothalamus-pituitary-testis axis, even when treated serum testosterone levels remain within the normal range.[34] Although cessation of short-term exogenous testosterone supplementation therapy usually results in recovery of spermatogenesis within several months, longer duration of therapy may impair spermatogenesis for 12 to 24 months or longer.[34,35]

Data suggest that a significant number of providers may not recognize the effects of testosterone on the hypothalamus-pituitary-testis axis. Of particular concern is a study that found 30% of practicing urologists reported prescribing testosterone as empirical therapy for idiopathic infertility.[36] Similarly, Samplaski and colleagues[37] reported that 1.3% of men presenting for infertility evaluation reported using testosterone, of which, 12% were prescribed testosterone specifically to treat their infertility. The average duration of use was 6 years, and 88% of the men were azoospermic. Of the men with no other identifiable cause of azoospermia, 65% recovered spermatogenesis within 6 months of discontinuing testosterone supplementation.[37]

TESTOSTERONE PRESCRIPTION ADHERENCE

The FDA reported that the average length of testosterone use was 6 months over the 5-year period analyzed.[11] Other studies, however, found increased rates of adherence. In one study, 66% of men with symptomatic testosterone deficiency remained on TST at 1 year.[22] This finding may be biased, however, as only men with symptoms and low testosterone levels were studied. Thus, men whose symptoms were not associated with testosterone deficiency and may not have improved with TST were not included in this study. Even after this caveat, 27% of the group discontinued therapy because of lack of clinical effectiveness, despite 97% having normalization of testosterone levels at 3 months.[22] Men with more severe symptoms were found to be more likely to continue therapy.[22] Another study from the United States found that only 30% of men with a diagnosis of hypogonadism who were prescribed topical TST adhered to their prescribed regimen, and only 20% continued TST for 12 months.[38] Among a similar population, 62% reported either temporarily or permanently discontinuing testosterone therapy, usually because of either cost or lack of effectiveness.[18] A follow-up study within this latter population found that adherence to nontopical, short-acting formulations was also low.[17] Finally, only 45% of a small cohort of Canadian men remained on TST 2 years after starting, with most men discontinuing because of lack of effectiveness.[39] Twenty-nine of the patients that discontinued use (representing 34% of the entire study group and 62% of the group that discontinued) had pretreatment testosterone levels within the normal range,[39] suggesting that symptoms in the absence of low testosterone may be less likely to respond to TST.

DIRECT-TO-CONSUMER PRODUCT ADVERTISING

Part of the public concern regarding the trends in the use of TST relates to direct-to-consumer product advertising and disease awareness communications. The effect of direct-to-consumer pharmaceutical advertising on health care is controversial.[40] Proponents argue that this advertising informs patients and empowers them to engage with physicians about health care issues that otherwise might go unaddressed. Critics contend that these advertisements result in overuse of newer drugs that are more expensive to the health care system and have unproven safety profiles. In 2010, the FDA sent a warning letter to one of the manufacturers of a testosterone product with regard to their internet Web site and promotional videos.[41] The letter stated that the promotional materials were misleading because they promoted unapproved uses of the product (ie, athletic performance enhancement), broadened the indication (ie, can be used to treat depression or sexual dysfunction), and overstated its efficacy. The company agreed to work with the FDA to alter their promotional materials.

Disease awareness communications are another means by which pharmaceutical companies can enhance demand for their products. These communications do not mention any specific drug and, thus, are not regulated by the FDA, although they are regulated by the Federal Trade Commission. Unfortunately, the symptoms of hypogonadism are nonspecific, which is why symptom-based screening instruments (eg, the Aging Deficiency in the Aging Male questionnaire) are not recommended.[30,42] The "Is It Low T?" campaign is among the most criticized disease awareness communications because of the nonspecific nature of the symptoms described and the implication that the relationship between hypogonadism and common comorbidities are

causal as opposed to associations.[43–45] Moreover, as the symptoms of low testosterone are not specific and are common among the aging population, this may lead to the belief that such symptoms are only caused by low testosterone. Indeed, a search for an elixir to counteract the declines in physical, sexual, and mental health associated with aging ultimately led to the discovery of testosterone (reviewed by Miller and Fulmer[46]). A formal complaint against these types of low testosterone campaigns was filed with Health Canada, which it rejected stating that such campaigns are not considered advertising.[47]

The dramatic increase in testosterone prescribing has evoked strong opinions regarding overprescribing on the one hand and criticism that not enough men with symptomatic testosterone deficiency are being treated on the other. Although the lay press has seized this controversy and published many articles, little scientific data exist regarding the public opinion of TST. A multitude of editorials and opinion pieces criticizing the increased trends in testosterone prescribing have been published in academic journals; a main focus of many of these articles are, again, the advertising practices of testosterone manufacturers.

Conversely, proponents of testosterone prescribing point to the number of men with symptomatic hypogonadism who do not receive therapy. For example, analysis of the Boston Area Community Health Survey participants found that 88% of men with symptoms and low testosterone levels (total testosterone <300 ng/dL and free testosterone <5 ng/dL) did not receive treatment.[48] Proponents of testosterone prescribing claim TST to be safe and point out weaknesses in the data on testosterone side effects and highlight studies showing a mortality benefit to testosterone supplementation therapy.[49–52]

Studies investigating the general public's opinions regarding TST are scarce. Two sources of information are available, however, including studies investigating subjects' attitudes toward the concept of LOH and attitudes toward anabolic androgenic steroids.

Several studies looked at how the general public understands and views the concept of LOH (referred to as *andropause* in these studies) and the source of information. A pilot study of 500 Chinese men found that although most were familiar with the concept of andropause, most felt it was a natural consequence of aging.[53] Mass media was the main source of information, and general understanding of the concept was poor.[53] In contrast, among men in Northern India, only 2.2% were familiar with the concept of andropause despite most of the subjects having symptoms of

LOH as measured with the Androgen Deficiency in the Aging Male (ADAM) questionnaire.[54] Only 11% were aware that treatment existed for the symptoms and 5.8% reported having taken testosterone. Although 47% would be willing to seek help for their symptoms, 33% reported they wouldn't take any treatment because they believed the symptoms were a natural part of aging and should not be treated.[54] A study of US men calling a medical information hotline to enquire about testosterone gel (around the time the gels were becoming available on the market) found that the primary care physician (47%) was the main source of clinical information, whereas the internet (52%) and popular press (18%) were the most frequent nonclinical sources of information.[55] More recent studies of North American or European men are not available.

FOOD AND DRUG ADMINISTRATION ACTIONS

Recent studies suggest a possible association between testosterone supplementation and cardiovascular risk.[56,57] These are reviewed extensively elsewhere in the issue (See Tanna MS, Schwartzbard A, Berger JS, et al: Management of hypogonadism in the cardiovascular patient: what are the implications of testosterone therapy on cardiovascular morbidity?, in this issue).

All studies have weaknesses that limit the conclusions that can be drawn from the data. Regardless of the criticisms levied against the methods of these articles, the authors' findings raised enough concern to initiate investigation by the FDA, the regulatory body responsible for safeguarding the US population from the adverse events of drugs.

In response to articles from Vigen and colleagues[56] and Finkle and colleagues,[57] the FDA released a Drug Safety Communication on January 31, 2014, stating that it was investigating the risk of stroke, heart attack, and death in men taking testosterone products.[58] The communication stated that the FDA had not yet concluded whether there was an increased risk of these cardiovascular events. The FDA did explicitly reinforce that testosterone products are only approved for use in men who have classic androgen deficiency owing to an associated medical condition such as a genetic condition or chemotherapy. Although not explicitly saying so, the language of the communication conveys that the FDA was not just concerned about the cardiovascular risk associated with testosterone use but also inappropriate use in men with LOH.

On September 17, 2014, the FDA's Center for Drug Evaluation and Research held a joint meeting with the Bone, Reproductive and Urologic Drugs Advisory and the Drug Safety and Risk Management Advisory Committees.[59] The objective was 2-fold: to identify the appropriate indicated population for TST and to assess whether there is a potential risk for major adverse cardiovascular events associated with testosterone use.

As a result of the Advisory Committee meeting, multiple changes were made to the labeling of testosterone products (**Fig. 1**).[60] The indications for the product previously included *idiopathic hypogonadotropic hypogonadism*; however, the panel felt that this term was vague enough that it could be interpreted to include LOH, which is often associated with a normal luteinizing hormone. By removing the term *idiopathic*, the panel hoped to reinforce the idea that TST is only appropriate for men who are hypogonadal owing to a well-defined cause such as Klinefelter's syndrome or pituitary tumor.

To further convey their concern regarding the overuse of testosterone therapy in men with LOH, the FDA also recommended additional language in the section regarding limitations of use. Previously, this section only stated that the safety and efficacy of testosterone therapy in boys younger than 18 years have not been established. The new label includes a similar statement regarding the use of testosterone therapy for men with age-related hypogonadism. Furthermore, language was added to the dose and administration instructions explicitly stating that men should have 2 separate morning serum testosterone values that are less than the normal range before initiating TST.

Finally, the FDA added language to the labeling stating their summary of the available literature concerning risk of cardiovascular events with the use of testosterone therapy. The label indicates that the studies are inconclusive as to whether there is an increased risk of myocardial infarction, nonfatal stroke, and cardiovascular death, but that some studies do show an increased risk of these events. The section concluded with the statement that patients should be informed about the possible risk.

The mandate of the FDA is to ensure that drugs sold to the public are efficacious and safe for use. Part of the impetus for the label changes on testosterone products is both their recognition of the trends in testosterone use and the cardiovascular safety concerns raised by certain studies. Although the organization cannot regulate how physicians and patients use these medications, the changes in the labeling make it explicitly clear that much of the use of testosterone is in an off-label form not sanctioned by the FDA.

INDICATIONS AND USAGE

Drug X is indicated for replacement therapy in adult males for conditions associated with a deficiency or absence of endogenous testosterone:

• Primary hypogonadism (congenital or acquired): testicular failure due to conditions such as cryptorchidism, bilateral torsion, orchitis, vanishing testis syndrome, orchiectomy, Klinefelter's syndrome, chemotherapy, or toxic damage from alcohol or heavy metals. These men usually have low serum testosterone concentrations and gonadotropins (follicle stimulating hormone [FSH], luteinizing hormone [LH]) above the normal range.

• Hypogonadotropic hypogonadism (congenital or acquired): idiopathic gonadotropin or luteinizing hormone-releasing hormone (LHRH) deficiency or pituitary-hypothalamic injury from tumors, trauma, or radiation. These men have low testosterone serum concentrations, but have gonadotropins in the normal or low range.

Limitations of use:

• Safety and efficacy of Drug X in men with "age-related hypogonadism" (also referred to as "late-onset hypogonadism") have not been established.

• Safety and efficacy of Drug X in males less than 18 years old have not been established.

• Topical testosterone products may have different doses, strengths or application instructions that may result in different systemic exposure.

DOSAGE AND ADMINISTRATION

Prior to initiating Drug X, confirm the diagnosis of hypogonadism by ensuring that serum testosterone concentrations have been measured in the morning on at least two separate days and that these serum testosterone concentrations are below the normal range.

WARNINGS AND PRECAUTIONS

Cardiovascular Risk

Long term clinical safety trials have not been conducted to assess the cardiovascular outcomes of testosterone replacement therapy in men. To date, epidemiologic studies and randomized controlled trials have been inconclusive for determining the risk of major adverse cardiovascular events (MACE), such as non-fatal myocardial infarction, non-fatal stroke, and cardiovascular death, with the use of testosterone compared to non-use. Some studies, but not all, have reported an increased risk of MACE in association with use of testosterone replacement therapy in men.

Patients should be informed of this possible risk when deciding whether to use or to continue to use Drug X.

Fig. 1. 2015 changes to testosterone product labels. (*From* United States Food and Drug Administration. FDA drug safety communication. 2015. Available at: http://www.fda.gov/Drugs/DrugSafety/ucm436259.htm. Accessed December 30, 2015.)

SUMMARY

TST has become increasingly popular since the turn of the century. Whether the increase in the use of these products is a result of increased recognition of a previously undiagnosed problem or the result of inappropriate marketing, misuse of the products remains controversial. Multiple studies suggest that testosterone products are prescribed in a manner inconsistent with medical organization guidelines. Although methodologically flawed, recent studies raised concern about cardiovascular risks associated with the use of TST. These concerns led the FDA to clarify the labeling of these products and request further research into potential cardiovascular effects associated with testosterone products. Results from these studies will help define the appropriate population for TST going forward. It is hoped that these data combined with physician and public education will minimize inappropriate prescribing and allow those likely to benefit from TST to receive it.

REFERENCES

1. Thompson WO. Uses and abuses of the male sex hormone. J Am Med Assoc 1946;132:185–8.
2. Morales A. The long and tortuous history of the discovery of testosterone and its clinical application. J Sex Med 2013;10(4):1178–83.
3. Institute of Medicine (US) Committee on Assessing the Need for Clinical Trials of Testosterone Replacement Therapy, Liverman CT, Blazer DG. Testosterone and aging: clinical research directions. Washington, DC: National Academies Press (US); 2004.
4. Layton JB, Li D, Meier CR, et al. Testosterone lab testing and initiation in the United Kingdom and the United States, 2000–2011. J Clin Endocrinol Metab 2014;99:835–42.
5. Baillargeon J, Urban RJ, Ottenbacher KJ, et al. Trends in androgen prescribing in the United States, 2001 to 2011. JAMA Intern Med 2013;173(15):1465–6.
6. Bhasin S, Singh AB, Mac RP, et al. Managing the risks of prostate disease during testosterone replacement therapy in older men: recommendations for a standardized monitoring plan. J Androl 2003;24(3):299–311.
7. Nguyen CP, Hirsch MS, Moeny D, et al. Testosterone and "Age-Related Hypogonadism"-FDA concerns. N Engl J Med 2015;373(8):689–91.
8. Jasuja GK, Bhasin S, Reisman JI, et al. Ascertainment of testosterone prescribing practices in the VA. Med Care 2015;53(9):746–52.
9. Handelsman DJ. Trends and regional differences in testosterone prescribing in Australia, 1991-2001. Med J Aust 2004;181(8):419–22.
10. Handelsman DJ. Global trends in testosterone prescribing, 2000-2011: expanding the spectrum of prescription drug misuse. Med J Aust 2013;199(8):548–51.

11. Mohamoud MA, Chai G, Staffa J. Drug use review. 412536 edition. n.d.

12. Piszczek J, Mamdani M, Antoniou T, et al. The impact of drug reimbursement policy on rates of testosterone replacement therapy among older men. PLoS One 2014;9(7):e98003.

13. Walsh TJ, Shores MM, Fox AE, et al. Recent trends in testosterone testing, low testosterone levels, and testosterone treatment among veterans. Andrology 2015;3(2):287–92.

14. Grossmann M, Anawalt BD, Wu FC. Clinical practice patterns in the assessment and management of low testosterone in men: an international survey of endocrinologists. Clin Endocrinol (Oxf) 2015; 82(2):234–41.

15. Behre HM, Christin-Maitre S, Morales AM, et al. Transversal European survey on testosterone deficiency diagnosis. Aging Male 2012;15(2):69–77.

16. Malik RD, Wang CE, Lapin B, et al. Characteristics of men undergoing testosterone replacement therapy and adherence to follow-up recommendations in metropolitan multicenter health care system. Urology 2015;85(6):1382–8.

17. Donatucci C, Cui Z, Fang Y, et al. Long-term treatment patterns of testosterone replacement medications. J Sex Med 2014;11(8):2092–9.

18. Shortridge EF, Polzer P, Donga P, et al. Experiences and treatment patterns of hypogonadal men in a U.S. health system. Int J Clin Pract 2014;68(10): 1257–63.

19. Katz A, Katz A, Burchill C. Androgen therapy: testing before prescribing and monitoring during therapy. Can Fam Physician 2007;53(11):1936–42.

20. Gooren LJ, Behre HM, Saad F, et al. Diagnosing and treating testosterone deficiency in different parts of the world. Results from global market research. Aging Male 2007;10(4):173–81.

21. Canup R, Bogenberger K, Attipoe S, et al. Trends in androgen prescriptions from military treatment facilities: 2007 to 2011. Mil Med 2015;180(7):728–31.

22. Rhoden EL, Morgentaler A. Symptomatic response rates to testosterone therapy and the likelihood of completing 12 months of therapy in clinical practice. J Sex Med 2010;7(1 Pt 1):277–83.

23. Feldman HA, Longcope C, Derby CA, et al. Age trends in the level of serum testosterone and other hormones in middle-aged men: longitudinal results from the Massachusetts male aging study. J Clin Endocrinol Metab 2002;87(2):589–98.

24. Harman SM, Metter EJ, Tobin JD, et al. Longitudinal effects of aging on serum total and free testosterone levels in healthy men. Baltimore longitudinal study of aging. J Clin Endocrinol Metab 2001;86(2):724–31.

25. Travison TG, Araujo AB, O'Donnell AB, et al. A population-level decline in serum testosterone levels in American men. J Clin Endocrinol Metab 2007;92(1):196–202.

26. Shi Z, Araujo AB, Martin S, et al. Longitudinal changes in testosterone over five years in community-dwelling men. J Clin Endocrinol Metab 2013;98(8):3289–97.

27. Bhasin S, Cunningham GR, Hayes FJ, et al. Testosterone therapy in men with androgen deficiency syndromes: an endocrine society clinical practice guideline. J Clin Endocrinol Metab 2010; 95:2536–59.

28. Wang C, Nieschlag E, Swerdloff R, et al. Investigation, treatment, and monitoring of late-onset hypogonadism in males: ISA, ISSAM, EAU, EAA, and ASA recommendations. J Androl 2009;30:1–9.

29. Nieschlag E, Swerdloff R, Behre HM, et al. Investigation, treatment, and monitoring of late-onset hypogonadism in males: ISA, ISSAM, and EAU recommendations. J Androl 2006;27(2):135–7.

30. Bhasin S, Cunningham GR, Hayes FJ, et al. Testosterone therapy in adult men with androgen deficiency syndromes: an endocrine society clinical practice guideline. J Clin Endocrinol Metab 2006; 91:1995–2010.

31. Baillargeon J, Urban RJ, Kuo YF, et al. Screening and monitoring in men prescribed testosterone therapy in the U.S., 2001-2010. Public Health Rep 2015; 130(2):143–52.

32. Muram D, Zhang X, Cui Z, et al. Use of hormone testing for the diagnosis and evaluation of male hypogonadism and monitoring of testosterone therapy: application of hormone testing guideline recommendations in clinical practice. J Sex Med 2015;12(9): 1886–94.

33. Gu Y, Liang X, Wu W, et al. Multicenter contraceptive efficacy trial of injectable testosterone undecanoate in Chinese men. J Clin Endocrinol Metab 2009;94(6): 1910–5.

34. Nieschlag E, Vorona E, Wenk M, et al. Hormonal male contraception in men with normal and subnormal semen parameters. Int J Androl 2011;34(6 Pt 1):556–67.

35. Liu PY, Swerdloff RS, Christenson PD, et al. Rate, extent, and modifiers of spermatogenic recovery after hormonal male contraception: an integrated analysis. Lancet 2006;367(9520):1412–20.

36. Ko EY, Siddiqi K, Brannigan RE, et al. Empirical medical therapy for idiopathic male infertility: a survey of the American urological association. J Urol 2012;187(3):973–8.

37. Samplaski MK, Loai Y, Wong K, et al. Testosterone use in the male infertility population: prescribing patterns and effects on semen and hormonal parameters. Fertil Steril 2014;101(1):64–9.

38. Schoenfeld MJ, Shortridge E, Cui Z, et al. Medication adherence and treatment patterns for hypogonadal patients treated with topical testosterone therapy: a retrospective medical claims analysis. J Sex Med 2013;10(5):1401–9.

39. McLaren D, Siemens DR, Izard J, et al. Clinical practice experience with testosterone treatment in men with testosterone deficiency syndrome. BJU Int 2008;102(9):1142–6.

40. Ventola CL. Direct-to-consumer pharmaceutical advertising: therapeutic or toxic? P T 2011;36(10): 669–84.

41. United States Food and Drug Administration. Warning letter to slate phamaceuticals. 2010.

42. Morley JE, Charlton E, Patrick P, et al. Validation of a screening questionnaire for androgen deficiency in aging males. Metabolism 2000;49(9):1239–42.

43. Schwartz LM, Woloshin S. Low "T" as in "template": how to sell disease. JAMA Intern Med 2013;173(15): 1460–2.

44. Gentry J, Price DJ, Peiris AN. Hypogonadism in primary care: the lowdown on low testosterone. South Med J 2013;106(9):492.

45. Perls T, Handelsman DJ. Disease mongering of age-associated declines in testosterone and growth hormone levels. J Am Geriatr Soc 2015;63(4):809–11.

46. Miller NL, Fulmer BR. Injection, ligation and transplantation: the search for the glandular fountain of youth. J Urol 2007;177(6):2000–5.

47. Eggertson L. Brouhaha erupts over testosterone-testing advertising campaign. CMAJ 2011;183: E1161–2.

48. Hall SA, Araujo AB, Esche GR, et al. Treatment of symptomatic androgen deficiency: results from the Boston area community health survey. Arch Intern Med 2008;168(10):1070–6.

49. Morgentaler A. Testosterone, cardiovascular risk, and hormonophobia. J Sex Med 2014;11(6):1362–6.

50. Shores MM, Matsumoto AM, Sloan KL, et al. Low serum testosterone and mortality in male veterans. Arch Intern Med 2006;166(15):1660–5.

51. Shores MM, Smith NL, Forsberg CW, et al. Testosterone treatment and mortality in men with low testosterone levels. J Clin Endocrinol Metab 2012; 97(6):2050–8.

52. Muraleedharan V, Marsh H, Kapoor D, et al. Testosterone deficiency is associated with increased risk of mortality and testosterone replacement improves survival in men with type 2 diabetes. Eur J Endocrinol 2013;169(6):725–33.

53. Yan YY. Awareness and knowledge of andropause among Chinese males in Hong Kong. Am J Mens Health 2010;4(3):231–6.

54. Ashat M, Puri S, Singh A, et al. Awareness of andropause in males: a North Indian study. Indian J Med Sci 2011;65(9):379–86.

55. Anderson JK, Faulkner S, Cranor C, et al. Andropause: knowledge and perceptions among the general public and health care professionals. J Gerontol A Biol Sci Med Sci 2002;57(12):M793–6.

56. Vigen R, O'Donnell CI, Barón AE, et al. Association of testosterone therapy with mortality, myocardial infarction, and stroke in men with low testosterone levels. JAMA 2013;310(17):1829–36.

57. Finkle WD, Greenland S, Ridgeway GK, et al. Increased risk of non-fatal myocardial infarction following testosterone therapy prescription in men. PLoS One 2014;9(1):e85805.

58. United States Food and Drug Administration. FDA drug safety communication: FDA evaluating risk of stroke, heart attack and death with FDA-approved testosterone products. 2014.

59. United States Food and Drug Administration. Joint meeting of the bone, reproductive and urologic drugs advisory committee (BRUDAC) and the drug safety and risk management advisory committee (DSaRM). 2014.

60. United States Food and Drug Administration. FDA drug safety communication. 2015.

Index

Urol Clin N Am 43 (2016) 273–277
http://dx.doi.org/10.1016/S0094-0143(16)00026-4
0094-0143/16/$ – see front matter © 2016 Elsevier Inc. All rights reserved.

Moving?

Make sure your subscription moves with you!

To notify us of your new address, find your **Clinics Account Number** (located on your mailing label above your name), and contact customer service at:

Email: journalscustomerservice-usa@elsevier.com

800-654-2452 (subscribers in the U.S. & Canada)
314-447-8871 (subscribers outside of the U.S. & Canada)

Fax number: 314-447-8029

Elsevier Health Sciences Division
Subscription Customer Service
3251 Riverport Lane
Maryland Heights, MO 63043

*To ensure uninterrupted delivery of your subscription, please notify us at least 4 weeks in advance of move.